Psychiatry and Technology

Scrivener Publishing
100 Cummings Center, Suite 541J
Beverly, MA 01915-6106

Publishers at Scrivener
Martin Scrivener (martin@scrivenerpublishing.com)
Phillip Carmical (pcarmical@scrivenerpublishing.com)

Psychiatry and Technology

Edited by

Raghavendra M. Devadas

Vani Hiremani

Preethi

Praveen Gujjar

Sapna R.

and

Manoj Shettar

Scrivener Publishing

WILEY

This edition first published 2026 by John Wiley & Sons, Inc., 111 River Street, Hoboken, NJ 07030, USA and Scrivener Publishing LLC, 100 Cummings Center, Suite 541J, Beverly, MA 01915, USA

For more information about Scrivener publications please visit www.scrivenerpublishing.com.

Wiley Global Headquarters
111 River Street, Hoboken, NJ 07030, USA

For details of our global editorial offices, customer services, and more information about Wiley products visit us at www.wiley.com.

The manufacturer's authorized representative according to the EU General Product Safety Regulation is Wiley-VCH GmbH, Boschstr. 12, 69469 Weinheim, Germany, e-mail: Product_Safety@wiley.com.

Library of Congress Cataloging-in-Publication Data

ISBN 9781394429639

Cover image: Generated with AI using Adobe Firefly
Cover design by Russell Richardson

Set in size of 11pt and Minion Pro by Manila Typesetting Company, Makati, Philippines

Printed in the USA

10 9 8 7 6 5 4 3 2 1

Contents

Preface

The discipline of Psychiatry has long stood at the intersection of mind, biology, and society, evolving in response to advances in neuroscience, psychology, and clinical practice. In recent years, a new and powerful force has begun to reshape this landscape: technology. The accelerating integration of digital tools, computational intelligence, and connected systems into mental health care marks a pivotal moment in the history of psychiatric science and practice. This book, *Psychiatry and Technology*, is conceived within this transformative context.

Technological innovation is no longer peripheral to psychiatry. Artificial intelligence, machine learning, telecommunication platforms, wearable sensors, virtual and augmented reality, and large-scale data analytics are increasingly influencing how mental health conditions are assessed, monitored, and treated. These developments are redefining clinical workflows, expanding access to care, and enabling more personalized and preventive approaches to mental health. At the same time, they raise profound questions regarding ethics, privacy, equity, clinical validity, and the evolving role of the mental health professional.

The purpose of this volume is to situate these technological advancements within the broader disciplinary evolution of psychiatry. Rather than presenting technology as a replacement for clinical judgment or human connection, the book approaches it as an enabling framework that has the potential to augment psychiatric insight, extend therapeutic reach, and support evidence-based decision-making. By examining both opportunities and limitations, the book seeks to foster a balanced and critical understanding of technology's role in mental health care.

Psychiatry and Technology bring together conceptual foundations, emerging methodologies, and future-oriented perspectives to illuminate how digital innovation is shaping contemporary and future psychiatric practice. It is intended to serve as a scholarly resource for clinicians, researchers, students, and technologists who seek to engage thoughtfully with this rapidly evolving field. In doing so, the book aspires to contribute to an informed, ethical, and human-centered integration of technology into psychiatry, aligned with the core mission of improving mental health outcomes across diverse populations.

Raghavendra M. Devadas
Vani Hiremani
Preethi
Praveen Gujjar
Sapna R.
and
Manoj Shettar

1

AI-Driven Innovations in Digital Psychiatry and Mental Health Ecosystems

Ameer Asra Ahmed[1]*, Vinish P.[1] and Harold Andrew Patrick[2]

[1]Department of Management Studies, Dayananda Sagar College of Arts, Science and Commerce, Bengaluru, India
[2]CMS Business School, Jain University, Bengaluru, India

Abstract
The COVID-19 pandemic has exacerbated the global mental health crisis, with India being a focal point. However, challenges persist, including social mistrust surrounding mental wellness, which fosters secrecy. A critical shortage of qualified mental health professionals exists, highlighted by current data showing that 8% of Indians suffer from mental health issues, straining the healthcare system. The psychiatrist-to-population ratio stands at only 0.75 per 100,000 people, resulting in lengthy wait times—urban patients may wait a year, whereas rural patients can wait 2 to 3 years. Vulnerable populations face unique biological, psychological, and socioeconomic risks, requiring tailored healthcare strategies. Additionally, environmental stressors contribute to increased mental health problems. Digital psychiatry is emerging as a transformative approach, integrating technology with traditional psychiatric methods. Mental health apps and telehealth services allow individuals to access care anytime and anywhere, overcoming previous barriers to treatment. However, these innovations should be implemented thoughtfully, addressing the specific challenges in mental healthcare. This paper aims to explore how technological advancements unfold amid ongoing hurdles faced in the development of digital psychiatry.

***Keywords*:** Mental health, digital psychiatry, mental health ecosystem, professional support, remote care, India

**Corresponding author*: azraahmed@dayanandasagar.edu

Raghavendra M. Devadas, Vani Hiremani, Preethi, Praveen Gujjar, Sapna R. and Manoj Shettar (eds.) Psychiatry and Technology, (1–28) © 2026 Scrivener Publishing LLC

1.1 Introduction

The global population experiences millions of cases of mental health issues. The scientific community has invested years of effort to establish multiple proven therapeutic approaches dealing with such issues. The COVID-19 epidemic disrupts medical services and adds extra stress to the population because many individuals face substantial barriers to receiving proper mental healthcare. Digital mental health services provided through mobile devices and online platforms improve access to care for various mental health interventions [1]. This allows great expansion of mental health service availability. People who reside in remote areas and regions lacking development can benefit from these services to remedy insufficient traditional care opportunities. Mental health interventions succeed when designers base their development including user-specific needs and implementation methods. Users need to be involved together with cultural relevance and pragmatic usability assessments to verify that these innovative opportunities serve everyone effectively. Herbal psychiatry uses modern technology and traditional psychiatric treatment to create a new approach that enhances diagnostic tools and prognostic methods for better therapy results in mental health treatment. Healthcare practitioners who use desktops, cell phones, laptops, and tablets are facilitating the digital transformation of psychiatry at this very moment. Digital devices help professionals perform crucial clinical responsibilities with better accuracy such as maintaining patient files and creating appointments and executing diagnosis assessments. Major advancements occur in mental healthcare because of technological solutions, which have recently emerged [2, 3]. Applications for mental health along with timely machine learning modules as well as real-time ecology evaluations that embrace both ancient practices and new technological implementations constitute current trial deployments. The technological innovations help mental health professionals diagnose and treat patients, yet represent a fundamental change in patient empowerment because they directly provide new mental health self-management tools to patients for more personalized healthcare services. The field of digital psychiatry advances rapidly by using present-day technology both to extend and in certain cases to replace traditional diagnostic procedures throughout mental health treatment. As an area of development, this sector brings together mobile apps and telehealth systems and specialized software dedicated to enhancing mental health service accessibility and quality. Several digital tools enable users to obtain healthcare information at any time from any location, thus resolving past practical and geographical limitations that posed treatment barriers [4]. Digital transformation stands as the fundamental factor that reduces diagnostic errors. Technology persists to track patient activities across time, which enables accurate data collection for clinicians to reduce mistakes coming from patient-reported wrong or selective information in office visits. This system prevents important information errors when such details should directly influence the diagnostic process and treatment approach. Digital psychiatry enables the capacity to preserve patient records whole for extensive periods of time. This digital storage maintains critical clinical information, which preserves main data while keeping it accessible for patients and healthcare providers through minimal deterioration. Converting healthcare practices to digital psychiatry proves challenging, even though there are certain benefits to this transition. The accuracy of reports generated through these techniques may suffer from device battery lifespan restrictions together with possible technical problems and calibration problems. While performing digital solutions with purpose and focus reduces connected dangers, health service providers need to maintain their technology and programs to achieve precise and dependable mental health treatment delivery.

1.2 Evolution of AI in Healthcare and Mental Health

Artificial intelligence (AI) has radically transformed healthcare, including mental health, over here, in the past few years. However, even as simple rule-based expert systems were used in the 1950s to support clinical decisions making, trips have never actually taken place.

Therefore, improving AI-assisted diagnosis and predictive analysis become possible with the appearance of machine learning techniques in the late 20th century, which first surfaced with the trend finding in big data. Through the 21st century, AI's applications in medicine were much deepened by deep learning, neural networks, and massive data processing. Figure 1.1 illustrates the evolution of AI in healthcare and mental health, from rule-based expert systems to advanced deep learning, AI-driven mental health tools, and future innovations such as brain–computer interfaces (BCIs) and real-time neural monitoring. These developments in mental health also led to greater efficiency and accessibility of AI-driven diagnostics and therapy recommendations alongside access to similar tailored patient management tools [5, 6].

AI has radically changed the mental health field, from basic chatbot models to advanced predictive analytics systems and therapy support apps. These AI tools use massive volumes of patient data: text therapy transcripts, speech patterns, and facial expressions, to precisely diagnose some mental health disorders such as depression, anxiety, and schizophrenia. Moreover, AI in medical procedures is

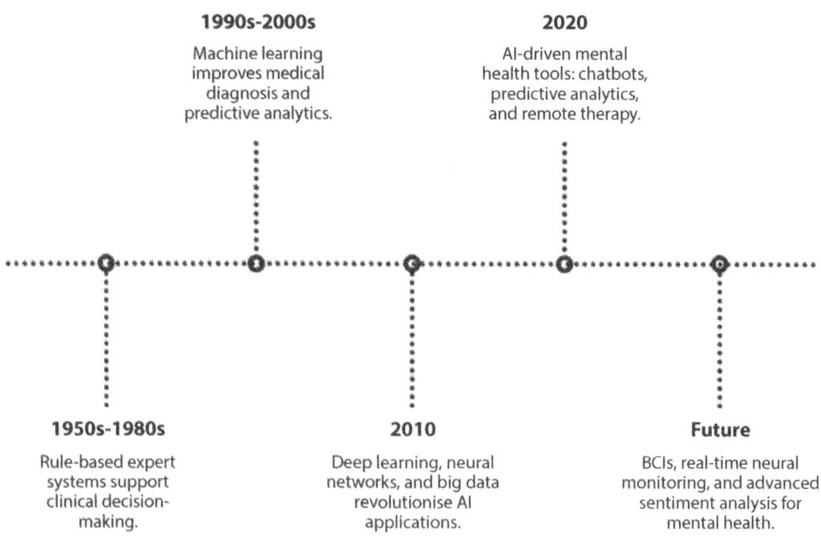

Figure 1.1 Evolution of AI in *healthcare* and *mental health*. Source: Authors.

getting more and more prevalent to track a patient's development, diagnose mental health issues, and adjust a therapy on the move. AI enhances available mental health professionals by facilitating better access, which in turn balances the needs of mental health professionals with the ability to visit the mental health institutions. AI digital systems enable remote consultations that break the barrier of distances and reduce wait times. Research using AI also assists in understanding of psychological and neurological diseases to provide more accurate and successful treatment plans.

The capacity of AI to monitor continuous data promotes a great change in psychiatry because of the possibility to find early warning of deterioration of mental health. In bipolar disease, AI can predict someone's likely severe depression, manic episodes, or suicidal thoughts by analyzing a person's online activity, speech patterns, wearable device inputs, and social media use. Early detection is vital because early detection helps to allow them to react in a timely fashion to stop crises before they get out of control. It is also noted that, as AI is improving, psychotherapy is as well, augmenting traditional means [7]. For maximum effectiveness of treatment, cognitive behavioral therapy (CBT) is combined in person with automated digital interventions with the help of AI. With virtual AI therapists, people's mental health can be aided by understanding the emotional context of that situation, as well as stimulating meaningful conversations and supporting the therapeutic guidance provided in a manner that is based on the principles of established psychology.

Yet, other important points persist regarding wider, general acceptance of AI in mental health. There are ethical questions, such as what happens to the data that the AI sees, whether an AI will have biases, and whether it would be a mistake not to trust human perception and concentration solely to AI. AI-based diagnosis and treatment plan are difficult or too difficult owing to the complexity of human emotions and the consciousness of mental health problems [8–10]. If AI and humans can maintain a balance, it will help so that AI does not replace humans when it comes to psychology. Because AI is growing quickly, its influence on mental health is likely to grow particularly through the invention of new technologies such as BCIs, real-time neural monitoring, and highly sophisticated sentiment analysis tools. Through continuous study and ethical debates, AI can provide more individualized and proactive, as well as globally accessible, solutions for mental health treatment.

1.3 Importance of Digital Psychiatry in Addressing Mental Health Challenges

In particular, mental health is extremely vital for digital psychiatry—this is the case for anyone in high-stress fields—information technology (IT) professionals, gig workers, night-shift employees, doctors, or nurses, all working on essential mental concerns. These groups face more demanding schedules and a higher degree of burnout, anxiety, and depression many times due to facing the demanding schedules and job uncertainty. Digital psychiatry tools such as online counseling services, self-help chatbot, or AI-powered therapy apps make mental health resources easy to access. This availability broadens well-being in general and contributes to lower the stigma [10]. What one can do with digital psychiatry is apply AI at a scale of needed treatment, at an individually tailored level, adjusted on different elements of many spheres. Moreover, apart from the personal mental health, digital psychiatry impacts workforce sustainability and organizational effectiveness. These are stress management strategy and real-time monitoring instruments, as well as AI-generated wellness programs for high-stress sectors. According to them, digital psychiatry also allows an early detection of psychological discomfort, which would allow companies to intervene earlier to build systems to reduce absenteeism and workplace burnout.

1.3.1 Rising Mental Health Challenges in High-Stress Jobs

Workers in high-stress fields mix long hours, job uncertainty, a mismatch between work and personal life, and heavy workloads. Some of these elements lead to major mental health problems such as depression, anxiety, burnout, and related psychiatric disorders [11–13]. Some types of workplace anxiety come with extremely negative effects on well-being. For example, IT workers have to sometimes produce outputs, often in the haste with high pressure. Anxiety, insomnia, and continual stress are caused by high production and unreasonable demands. Long hours in front of a screen are especially difficult for many IT experts, which aggravates mental and physical tiredness. This stress heightens as the sector operates at a fast pace, although job instability can aggravate matters (at times) [14].

Gen Z employees also have a particular problem in navigating a fast-changing employment environment. The pressure of social media has its toll, and then there are society expectations that are yet to be realized, which then often leads to more anxiety and stress as a result of the need for steady work. According to some studies, so many young people suffer from mental health problems due to loneliness and financial instability. It is in a job market that performance and competitiveness are at the forefront of forcing their emotional load forward [15, 16]. So, gig workers (freelancers and contractors) deal with a lot of difficulties because they are dealing with an inherent uncertainty of their job. Chronic stress, anxiety, and depression worsen when there is absence of job security, irregular income, and lack of occupational support systems. These workers are not full-time employees—and therefore usually absent access to mental health benefits offered by their companies. It puts them on a cycle of pressure, compromising their general welfare while they are unrelenting with their hunt of new ideas. This is particularly the case for night shift workers in manufacturing (and other industries) who will have disrupted circadian rhythms, thus increasing the risk depression, anxiety, insomnia, and mood swings. Some studies claim that synthetic work hours disrupt their ability to keep up with a sleep schedule as they have tiredness, poor attention, and emotional instability because of them [17, 18]. Over time, then, the totality of sleep issues can turn into a major hindrance to cognitive as well as physical health. Despite them being at the frontlines of healthcare, nurses and doctors often forfeit their mental health to accommodate

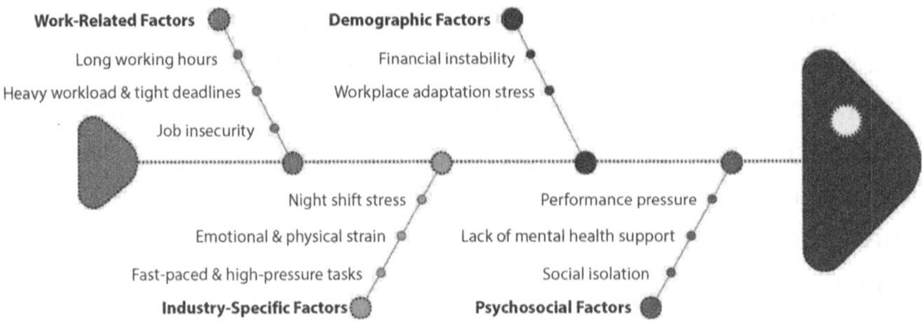

Figure 1.2 Fishbone *diagram*: causes of mental health challenges in high-stress jobs. Source: Authors.

the healthy, demanding nature of their work. There are some measures through which long hours, exposure to medical emergencies, the emotional toll of working with seriously ill patients, and high workplace pressure lead to burnout, posttraumatic stress disorder (PTSD), and depression. Even while delivering patient care, many medical practitioners work under lots of stress, sometimes even to the point of putting their own health on second thought. In addition, medical professionals have a stigma related to mental health problem that prevents professionals from getting necessary help. Figure 1.2 illustrates the key contributors to mental health challenges in high-stress jobs, categorizing them into work-related, industry-specific, demographic, and psychosocial factors.

Overall, the high-stress industries are progressively taxing employees with mental health issues. What digital psychiatry and AI can do is provide easily available, efficient mental health support to people in these hectic fields.

1.3.2 How Digital Psychiatry Addresses These Challenges

Due to the delivery of mental health treatment especially for employees in demanding environments, digital psychiatry is revolutionizing mental health treatment. Digital psychiatry delivers the same mental health support quick and easily available as one that you get by AI, telemedicine, and data analytics. It is especially helpful to those who might otherwise have a hard time obtaining traditional mental health services because of stigma, time limits, or plain place [19, 20]. One of the big advantages of digital psychiatry is that the supply of mental health support can be anywhere, at any time. AI-powered chatbots and digital therapists offer round-the-clock help in light of the fact that workers can instantly access assistance; they no longer have to wait for an appointment [21, 22]. With telepsychiatry systems, even more access is improved by allowing people to talk to licensed mental health professionals remotely [23, 24]. This will also be very helpful for gig workers, night shift workers, and IT professionals with a haphazard schedule, for instance, and perhaps difficulty attending conventional therapy sessions.

Digital psychiatry goes beyond that, as another key part of it is individualized treatment. In AI-driven platforms, AI searches patterns in how someone speaks, mental health, and psychological data to offer custom advice therapy. In addition, these sites also offer self-help materials, guided mindfulness activities, and CBT programs that employees might use at their own pace. Thus, such personalization promises people the most appropriate mental health support based on their own requirements [25, 26]. Mostly, help prevents worsening of mental health problems if recognized and if intervened early. Wearable technology helps track indicators of wellness such as heart rate variations, stress, and sleep cycles and then provides insights on a person's mental wellness. These technologies make it possible to early identify mental health issues so that they can lead to speedy treatment before the situation gets worse. For example, human resources departments or mental health experts could use predictive analytics to find workers who might be suffering from burnout or depression so that the respective support systems could be enabled [27, 28].

Digital psychiatry looks more and more like a part of the corporate mental health programs, and they are trying to raise employee well-being. AI-driven wellness apps allow companies to monitor the mental health of their staff and go ahead with specific mental health initiatives. Absolutely crucial to the health of a company is digital employee assistance programs, which offer resilience training, stress management seminars, and confidential counseling [29, 30]. Using these tools, high-stress sectors such as IT and healthcare can make good work environments with high mental health in mind.

One area where digital psychiatry is rather important is in resolving the stigma regarding mental health. For fear that their colleagues or supervisors will criticize them, many workers are reluctant to ask for help. AI-driven platforms have self-assessment tools and the anonymous mental health screening that gives people a way to assess their mental health without the need for any dependence on a third party. Additionally, AI-based sentiment analysis tools can gauge not only the emotions, but also stress in workplace communication, so that companies can help with things workers might not want to speak about out loud. Digital psychiatry also enhances the overall treatment by stressing on work–life balance and stress management. AI-driven wellness apps give time management techniques, guided meditation sessions, and relaxation activities to allow workers to take responsibility of their stress in a proper way. To ensure staff members practice self-care all through the working day, certain systems send reminders for breaks, hydration, and physical activity [31].

Particularly helpful to them will be these digital tools, because of professionals working in conditions with high demand, where burnout is one of the things these professionals encounter. Elsewhere, digital psychiatry will increasingly be required for occupational mental health. Future possible advancement can be emotional intelligence coaching by AI for managers to help them support their teams. Automatically changing lighting, ambiance, and workload distribution might create a more psychologically favorable work environment in stress-sensitive smart work environments. For instance, AI mental health assistants embedded into virtual collaboration tools would likely provide on demand emotional support to employees who are likely to make them feel heard and appreciated [32, 33]. In the end, digital psychiatry is changing how mental health treatment is ultimately delivered, through greater accessibility, an approach that utilizes a proactive method of care, and a personalized method of care. To better support companies' workers dealing with issues of their mental health, integrating wearable technology, predictive analytics, telepsychiatry, and AI-driven solutions will be helpful. Nowadays, employees are facing increasing mental health issues, and the solution for them will be integrating AI in mental health strategies as technology develops.

1.3.3 Future of Digital Psychiatry in Workplace Mental Health

Fast developments in digital technologies and AI offer digital psychiatry in corporate mental health interesting future opportunities. AI-driven mental health solutions are expected to provide more customized and proactive support to workers [34, 35]. Combining AI with digital psychiatry, we can continuously track mental health and use that real-time data analysis so as to start early interventions and create more effective treatment strategies. Digital psychiatry has advanced due to the improvement in emotional intelligence due to AI. The future AI systems that will be able to understand more complicated emotional expressions and the behavioral pattern will have deeper mental state knowledge. Doing so will close the gap between virtual mental health assistance provided by AI and human therapy and allow virtual mental health assistants to have more meaningful and sympathetic interactions.

Besides that, biometric data from wearable devices and Internet of Things (IoT)–equipped workspaces with AI-powered stress detection systems would probably be integrated into workplace environment. They will analyze several other stress indicators such as skin conductivity and typing speed and will try to spot early burnout or emotional discomfort [36, 37]. Therefore, companies will be able to deploy timely interventions to ease stress: including tailored wellness programs, changes in workload, or motivating breaks. Predictive analytics driven by AI will also be very important in determining the direction of occupational mental health. A behavior record can contain everything from how long you sleep, frequency of exercise, the food you ate, the apps you used, and more that can be extracted and processed by AI models to effectively predict mental health risk and thus predict workers who might be silently experiencing severe anxiety, depression, or burnout before disabling symptoms set in. There may be such proactive steps such as reducing absenteeism, increasing job satisfaction, and better working conditions.

Another interesting field of interest was the development of AI-powered emotional support systems that were, in fact, put inside business cooperation tools. These AI mental health assistants will set their eyes within the digital communication platforms at real-time emotional or stress [38]. Quick coping strategies, mindfulness practices, and gotchas to looking for professional help where required will be offered to give continuous mental health support during the working day.

Also, AI-driven workplace wellness programs are going to become much more advanced. Digital psychiatry platforms will consider the work schedule, stress levels, and personal circumstances of their employees and will offer a tailor-made mental plan, which is adapted to meet specific employee needs [39]. These platforms might also have gamified mental health activities, online support groups, and AI-guided therapy sessions that make staff members involved in their mental wellness path. The digital psychiatry in the workplace, at last, will finally make ethical concerns and data privacy a priority in its growth. As AI starts to play a role in mental health treatment, security and confidentiality of employee data will become important. For companies and AI creators, maintaining trust and silencing the use of private mental health data depend on their following rigorous ethical standards and data security policies [40].

1.4 AI-Powered Mental Health Tools: The Role of Chatbots and Virtual Therapists

Virtual therapists, self-assessment apps, and chatbots that use AI are some mental health tools. Woebot and Wysa are examples of such chatbots that provide CBT interventions by giving immediate emotional support. VR exposure therapy is being used to treat both PTSD and anxiety. AI-powered sentiment analysis tools help us to assess a person's emotional status and provide early intervention chances using the text and voice inputs. Such instruments ensure anonymity, which strengthens the availability and the cost of mental health treatment [41].

Mental health technologies will develop to enhance psychological assessment, as AI takes on role in influencing AI mood tracking, emotional prediction, and speech pattern analysis on digital platforms. The development of these systems improves the effectiveness of digital therapy through real-time emotional feedback and therefore customized treatments. Moreover, mental health tools connect with electronic health records (EHRs) in increasingly diverse ways so that medical practitioners can gain a full picture of patient history and treatment outcomes [42].

With the evolution of digital psychiatry, the tools of AI incorporating increasing amount of involvement for mental health came to become indispensable in the psychological support systems of the present time. Decreased stigma, improved convenience and access, and affordability are changing the access care by introduction of AI virtual therapists, chatbots, and mental health apps.

The use of AI-powered mental health tools is widespread, and chatbots are one of them. But these virtual assistants are real-time psychological assistance and guidance along with therapy. Chatbots use natural language processing (NLP) to text-based interaction with users by offering empathy, suggesting coping mechanisms, guiding people through evidence-based therapeutic activities such as CBT, and so having text-based interactions with users. Chatbot interventions such as Woebot and Wysa demonstrate that chatbots are extremely effective at lowering depression, anxiety, and stress symptoms.

This is unique as it differs from conventional therapy where users can receive help whenever they need it, through chatbots without scheduling anything. This will be particularly helpful for those whose social anxiety or stigma prevents them from approaching human therapists. AI chatbots are able to provide personalized treatments by continuously collecting data about their users. Chatbots are not all that is developing when it comes to AI virtual therapists. To provide personalized emotional support, they use sentiment analysis, facial expression analysis, and voice recognition [43]. They include some AI systems, which can suggest apt mental health resources and can listen to your mood swings by listening to speech patterns.

In addition, digital mental health tools have mobile apps with AI that deliver therapeutic programs. These apps contain usually guided meditation, stress management strategies, mood tracking, and self-help tools to empower the consumers on the way of their mental health. AI-based applications can analyses user behavior, identify the pattern of distress, and suggest mental health improvement. AI-enhanced mental health tools—virtual therapists and chatbots—have been making their way into increasing access and personalization, which is changing the mental healthcare scene. In so far as these technologies progress further, they will help make efficient mental health treatments accessible in many spheres and fields ranging from many ordinary professions.

1.5 Wearable Devices and IoT for Early Detection of Mental Health Conditions

Smartwatches and other wearable devices such as health monitors that are IoT compatible are used for early detection of mental health issues. Physiological signals of heart rate variability, sleep patterns, and physical activity related to mental health problems such as depression and anxiety, as well as AI surveillance for early warning signals, are also monitored in an effort to facilitate preventive effort. By working together, AI and wearables improve real-time monitoring and predictive functions, thus allowing doctors to offer fast response and an effective support. Beyond physiological monitoring, wearable technologies are on the verge of integration of voice and facial recognition technologies assessing the emotional condition [44]. These devices will now track fluctuations in tone of voice, expressions, and patterns of breathing, pointing up feelings of discomfort. All this comprehensive approach does heighten the whole mental health an individual has and brings the diagnosis accuracy level to a high bid. This allows one to safely combine wearables with AI-based therapeutic tools that can provide immediate response with guided meditations and stress-relieving activities to assist at real-time symptom relief [45].

Continuous tracking of the physiological and behavioral signal has been transformed by wearable devices and the IoT. Real-time data of variables such as heart rate variability, sleep quality, physical activity, and stress levels are collected by smartwatches, fitness trackers, and biosensors that supply perceptive analysis of a person's mental state. These tools mainly allow for the detection of early stages of deterioration in the mental health scenario to enable interventions before the condition turns serious [46, 47]. In addition to wearables, IoT devices should be incorporated in mental health treatment. Health devices that are linked, voice assistant devices, and smart home devices can all monitor changes in behavior, changes in the pitch of someone's voice, and small signals indicating that someone may be showing signs of social withdrawal, that is, mental health issues. Featuring IoT-driven devices guarantees proper connection with the healthcare providers for remote monitoring and quick help if required. AI-powered analytics also sieve massive data from these devices to find out the connected trend to depression, anxiety, and other psychological diseases. One of the advantages of wearable technology is that it is able to give people insights tailored to their mental health. They would be fed guided relaxation suggestions, real-time notifications, and stress-relieving techniques integrating with their physiological readers. This proactive method enables persons to manage their mental health, thus reducing their need for traditional modes of therapy. To be able to have ethical and efficient usage of wearable and IoT-based mental health solutions, there need to be resolved problems of security of data and potential bias in AI assessment, and legislative action is required. Because new technology for early identification, intervention, and treatment within mental healthcare will become more important with technology development, it will be using wearable devices and IoT. They have the realization to transform quality of life for a plethora of people from various backgrounds, through the use of these advances that can be made to make mental health treatment more customized, more accessible, and more preventive.

1.6 Role of AI in Predictive Analysis

One way that AI is speciating mental health treatment is using predictive analytics to spot people at risk for disorders such as depression or suicide. These analytics, powered by machine learning, analyse countless data points such as social media behavior, wearable technology data and EHRs to predict potential mental health crises. AI suicide risk assessment tools help doctors more effectively identify those who are at especially high risk, so that they can provide quick interventions aimed at saving lives. When we include AI in mental health projections, a data-centric way to predictive treatment is uncovered. Deep learning methods are being applied to these models to identify what are these minute trends that convey that the mental health of the world is declining. Through thorough behavioral data over time, AI can find deviations from normal psychological functioning [48–50]. These insights produce early warnings so that mental health treatment becomes proactive instead of reactive.

AI-based predictive analytics is transforming mental healthcare by way of early identification and intervention for some of the psychological disorders. Machine learning algorithms take an excruciating look at buckets upon buckets of patient data—the words they talk, the tweets they tweet, their biometric data, and medical histories—to identify potential anxiety and suicidal ideation risks. AI can pick up on subtle trends that human practitioners may miss; therefore, it can support early intervention and improve the accuracy of one's mental health assessment [51]. Suicide prevention is among the applications of predictive analytics in psychiatry because AI psychiatric models can predict behaviors of suicidal subjecting to factors of risk, such as a language, social disengagement, and unusual sleep patterns. Having AI in the mental health helplines and crisis intervention programs means experts are actively involved to help people while their crises are still not too serious.

In addition, AI is able to make individualized treatment plans because it watches patient response to treatments all the time. Predictive models predict individual responses to different treatments and recommend the best course of action this time [51]. Similarly, sentiment analysis powered by AI also analyzes voice and text communication to let doctors regularly monitor the emotional well-being of the patients and have real-time patient mental health analysis.

Moral questions do pop up in respect to predictive analytics' application in mental health treatment, such as algorithmic bias and data privacy. AI models need to be built using different datasets with precautions for ethical uses, and they should underline open decision-making. As AI progresses in areas such as first detection, personalized treatment, and proactive mental health strategies, predictive analytics will become increasingly important, and it will benefit us to improve access and effectiveness of mental healthcare.

1.7 AI-Powered Social Media and Sentiment Analysis

Social media has become the center of life and your relationship, your ideas, and your health. These sites can compromise mental health and cause articles of cyberbullying, social comparison, and exposure to upsetting content, while providing opportunities to take an active part in the community and express themselves.

AI-enabled emotional sentiment analysis has brought some fresh interesting take on community and personal mental health, which can be considered something that has emerged recently. Sentiment analysis, also referred to as opinion mining, is a methodology by which AI and NLP can be used to comprehend, categorize, and evaluate an expressed emotion in text. There is also an enormous amount of data that people comment, post, and interact on social media that can be assessed to determine trends in psychological stress, mood, and the development of mental health problems. An AI model looks at language, emoji's, tone, and context to determine if the material being assessed conveys a positive emotional impact, a neutral emotional impact, or a negative emotional impact. In that sense, this capacity is helpful to companies, mental health experts, and researchers to be able to more accurately identify people likely to have mental health issues and address broader mental health problems.

The most important use of AI aided by sentiment analyzing is to prevent suicide. Many people in crisis first chat with the emotions they hold on to social media before consulting experts. As an example, AI systems that use language markers of suicidal thoughts, such as expressions of hopelessness, self-harm, or withdrawal from social events, can alert humans about troubling posts. The AI algorithms used to identify possibly suicidal material and notify crisis intervention teams include Facebook and Twitter [52, 53]. These AI systems provide early warnings, which gives support networks the opportunity to intervene before things spin out of control, thus potentially saving lives.

Sentiment analysis that is motivated by AI is furthermore very helpful in identifying anxiety and depression. Some studies have shown that people suffering from mental issues might exhibit minor but consistent changes in engagement, writing style, or subjects of writing whenever they were online [54, 55]. These behavioral patterns can be tracked over time by the AI models that help the mental health professionals to remotely evaluate the emotional well-being. Some mental health apps now include sentiment analysis into their products to provide consumers with tailored insight on their emotions based on their social media activity.

Sentiment analysis powered by AI will help one to understand more general society mental health trends rather than being confined to personal assessments. Through complete statistical evaluation of social media sites, investigators can interrogate how crowded is the crowd on important concerns encompassing political turmoil, economic crisis, and health crisis. For example, during the COVID-19 epidemic, AI tools have also been used to help track, as well as combat, risk of collective anxiety and depression levels in different areas, to be available not only to mental health organizations but also in the distribution of resources for legislators.

It is combatting online toxicity, another absolutely vital use of AI in social media research. Cyberbullying, harassment, and the spread of negative content can take a serious-enough toll on mental health especially among younger users. AI-powered content moderation systems look for negative language and flag abusive messages and cutback of damaging contents. Online cyberbullying is an issue that websites such as YouTube, Instagram, and TikHub try to detect and prevent them through the sentiment analyzer [56].

Even so, there are ethical and privacy questions that sentiment analysis from AI raises. Surveillance of social media activity may violate user's permission and security. Also, AI models may have prejudices and would therefore interpret sarcasm, slang, or reference to culture wrong and evaluate them incorrectly. For AI to be used to support mental health, there need to be clear policies and ethical frameworks to balance the use of the technology with the protection of user privacy [4, 49, 52].

In the end, AI-driven sentiment analysis has enormous opportunity to improve mental health treatment. I think that AI is changing the second way people look at emotional well-being in an increasingly digital age by providing real-time insights, better knowledge of more general mental health trends, and the ability to identify the risks more easily. As AI models continue to grow and develop more sophisticated methods of inclusion into mental healthcare, mental healthcare will shift to a more proactive and responsive model that will help to support mental health support [33].

1.8 Mental Health Ecosystem in India

Digital psychiatry and AI change the mental health scene of India. We are experiencing a grossly high shortage in mental health professionals in the nation, and AI-driven solutions are the only means to bridge the treatment gap. Efforts in telepsychiatry, AI-based mental health apps, and other government-sponsored digital health projects, among others, are helping to improve access to treatment. And yet there remain issues of society stigma, poor digital literacy, and legal barriers if AI is to be most effective in helping India's mental health scene. Digital psychiatry has the potential to improve mental health treatments, providing them for people all around through making it more accessible, customized, and effective by leveraging AI. The changing mental health framework of the nation is being driven by a mixture of policy changes, technical developments, and AI-enhanced applications created to meet India's immediate mental health needs. Figure 1.3 illustrates the framework of AI in the mental health ecosystem in India, highlighting the integration of AI across various facets of mental healthcare. Despite growing awareness of it, India still suffers a mental health crisis that takes place in the realm of stigma, poor infrastructure, and an absolute dearth of qualified professionals. The Mental Healthcare Act (2017) and the National Mental Health Program together provide formidable legal

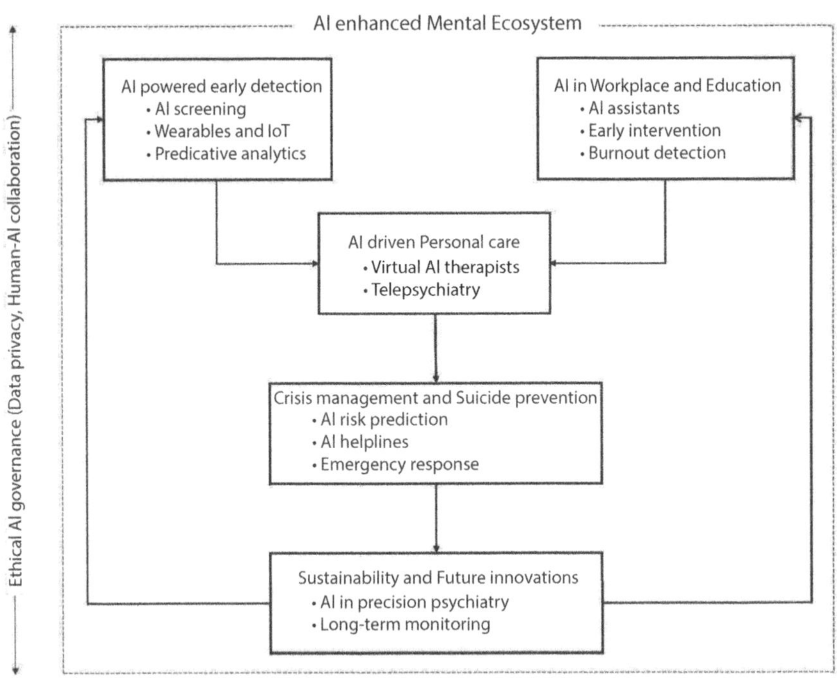

Figure 1.3 Framework of AI in mental health ecosystem in India. Source: Authors.

and structural foundations, which ensure adequate mental health services by and for a larger population. Yet, there is massive difference in access and gaps in implementation that remain the main obstacles, especially in rural areas [17, 43]. Digital mental health solutions have been one of the innovative answers to these problems. Of course, remote consultation, thanks to the development of telepsychiatry, has facilitated lowering of reliance on facilities and the accessibility of mental health treatments in "less privileged" areas. Chatbots AI-powered as well as mobile applications in mental health provide much more coverage in range of mental healthcare in terms that they can give immediate help and course of depression, anxiety, and other psychological conditions [31, 47]. National digital mental health solutions make way forward in the form of initiatives beginning from the Indian government such as the MANAS app. The way India's mental health landscape is changing is as digital psychological methods and AI go all in together.

AI-driven mental health diagnostics, predictive analysis, therapy support tools are gaining importance day by day. This way AI can analyze social media activity, text-based communication, or speech patterns to find out early symptoms of mental health so that it can help in timely intervention. Sentiment analysis powered by AI has been used to monitor public mental health trends in India to monitor the situation, thus allowing the legislators and mental health agencies to allocate resources efficiently [12, 44].

However, there are many ethical and logistical questions to be raised concerning that AI in India's mental health scene [18, 53]. If we want to be sure that AI-based solutions for mental health are equitable and work, there are issues to resolve: data security, privacy, and algorithmic biases. Additionally, the gap of the digital gap is still a key problem, as there are many people in the remote and economically underdeveloped areas who do not have access to smartphones and internet, in turn diminishing their chances of getting a benefit from digital mental health treatments [5, 46]. Going ahead, India's mental health system will need to harmonically integrate human led psychiatric treatment with technology. Although digital tools and AI can help increase early identification and increase accessibility, they cannot substitute for empathy and such a rich understanding that is provided by licensed mental health professionals [39]. To create a more inclusive, meaningful, and ethical mental health environment in India, it requires a partnership where AI would help to supplement as opposed to replace human know-how.

1.9 Conclusion

AI is transforming the digital psychiatry by bringing much improved accessibility, personalization, and overall efficacy of mental health treatment. More access is among the most obvious advantages of AI. These AI-driven tools such as digital counselors, chatbots, and telepsychiatrists take out the location specific hurdles across financial as well as social barriers so that even psychological support is offered in far-off places. This ensures that people could get the care that they require, even though in a case of a lack of specialists within their locale. Unlike these traditional therapies, with their scheduled appointments and covered schedules, these AI resources are freely usable 24/7 so as to avoid letting people down in places and even when they need it. On top of that, AI NLP capabilities are able to break through the barriers caused by culture and language in mental healthcare and promote inclusiveness. AI also personalizes that mental health treatment through customizing interventions to match certain needs. AI systems examine user data, including speech patterns, mood swings, and behavioral changes to develop tailor-made therapy recommendations. Also, by means of such dynamic learning, they change their responses in response to ongoing conversations with the user, thus ensuring the support is relevant and customized. Additionally, AI can intervene quickly with predictive analytics identifying small changes of behavior related to the onset of the mental health issue. Consequently, AI understands emotional states and offers real-time strategies for coping, all of which enables text, voice, and face expression to be analyzed using the sentiment analysis tools for aiding the mental health treatment to be more dynamic and effective.

It enables providers and patients to have data-driven insights into mental health treatment, making AI contribute to the enhancing the general efficacy of mental health treatment. The principal applications of the advanced AI diagnostic tools involve early identification of disorders such as depression, anxiety, and PTSD on the basis of trends in speech, writing, and behavior associated with these disorders. AI also aids medical professionals to reinforce how clinical judgment ought to be done, by analyzing huge volumes of data and being able to suggest evidence-based treatment routes. Such technologies consist of wearable technologies linked with AI that track stress levels, heart rate, and sleep patterns, giving instantaneous feedback on the mental health of each person.

The main benefit for digital psychiatry is that AI is capable of creating stigma-free environments in which the people can anonymously seek treatment. It decreases anxiety of judgment, making mental healthcare more accessible to a larger population. This, however, does not come without its difficulties on the side of AI-based digital psychiatry. First priority is to maintain patient records after breach and confidentiality. AI algorithms need to be taught on different datasets so that they are not exposed to reputations that might lead to a recommendation of erroneous or unfair treatment. Even when AI can help a great deal, there is nothing it can do to substitute emotional understanding and empathy of the human therapist. In fact, such a combination of AI's advantages with traditional psychiatric treatment is therefore mandatory.

AI will certainly raise accessibility, efficiency, and proactivity and allow it to significantly and positively influence mental health treatment. If they are still difficult to ensure AI is used in a continuous investigation and in an ethical usage, even in this context, AI is likely to become useful rather than substitute human-driven psychological therapy. Digital psychiatry will continue advancing and improving mental health outcomes everywhere with sense application of AI technologies.

AI disclosure statement: The author acknowledges the use of AI-based tools for minor language editing or grammatical correction. However, all intellectual contributions, analyses, and conclusions presented in this chapter are entirely the author's own.

References

1. Abbott, R., The Legal and Ethical Challenges of AI in Mental Health Care, Cambridge University Press, 2022.
2. Adams, S., Brown, T., Clark, L., Artificial Intelligence in Mental Health: Innovations and Implications, Oxford University Press, 2023.
3. American Psychiatric Association, AI and Psychiatry: The Future of Digital Mental Health Care, APA Publishing, Washington, DC, 2020.
4. Andrews, G., Basu, A., Cuijpers, P., Craske, M.G., McEvoy, P., English, C.L., Computer therapy for the anxiety and depression disorders is effective, acceptable and practical health care: An updated meta-analysis. *J. Anxiety Disord.*, 55, 70–78, 2018, doi:10.1016/j.janxdis.2018.01.001.
5. Banerjee, D. and Nair, V.S., Digital mental health and COVID-19: Using technology to scale up mental health services for India. *Asian J. Psychiatry*, 54, 102275, 2020, doi:10.1016/j.ajp.2020.102275.
6. Ben-Zeev, D., Digital mental health and AI: A revolution in psychiatric care. *Lancet Psychiatry*, 7, 5, 377–380, 2020, doi:10.1016/S2215-0366(20)30087-9.
7. Bickmore, T.W., Puskar, K., Schlenk, E.A., Pfeifer, L.M., Sereika, S.M., Maintaining reality: The role of conversational agents in mental health support. *J. Med. Internet Res.*, 21, 5, e12520, 2019, doi:10.2196/12520.
8. Brennan, K., Phan, T., Lohn, A., Ethical implications of AI-driven mental health monitoring. *AI Soc.*, 37, 3, 415–428, 2022, doi:10.1007/s00146-021-01176-w.
9. Bucci, S., Schwannauer, M., Berry, N., The digital revolution and its impact on mental health care. *Natl. Hum. Behav.*, 3, 2, 109–110, 2019, doi:10.1038/s41562-018-0491-5.
10. Bzdok, D. and Meyer-Lindenberg, A., Machine learning for precision psychiatry: Opportunities and challenges. *Biol. Psychiatry Cognit. Neurosci. Neuroimaging*, 3, 3, 223–230, 2018, doi:10.1016/j.bpsc.2018.01.003.

11. Carr, S., AI in mental health: The promise and perils of digital psychiatry. *Lancet Digit. Health*, 2, 2, e62–e63, 2020, doi:10.1016/S2589-7500(20)30003-7.
12. Chakrabarti, S. and Kaur, H., Machine learning in psychiatry: A new era in mental health research in India. *Indian J. Psychol. Med.*, 41, 6, 511–517, 2019, doi:10.4103/IJPSYM.IJPSYM_203_19.
13. Christodoulou, J.A. and Silver, C.H., AI-enhanced neuropsychological assessment: A new frontier in mental health diagnostics. *Neuropsychol. Rev.*, 32, 1, 67–81, 2022, doi:10.1007/s11065-021-09510-6.
14. Cowls, J. and Floridi, L., Prolegomena to a white paper on digital psychiatry ethics. *Philos. Technol.*, 31, 4, 503–525, 2018, doi:10.1007/s13347-018-0316-5.
15. Darcy, A.M., Louie, A.K., Roberts, L.W., Machine learning and the profession of medicine. *JAMA*, 315, 6, 551–552, 2016, doi:10.1001/jama.2015.18421.
16. DelPozo-Banos, M., *et al.*, Predicting suicidal risk using machine learning and electronic health records. *Transl. Psychiatry*, 11, 69, 2021, doi:10.1038/s41398-020-01117-8.
17. Doraiswamy, P.M. and Narayanan, S., Artificial Intelligence in Mental Health Care: Transforming Diagnosis and Treatment in India, AIIMS Publications, New Delhi, 2023.
18. Desai, G. and Chaturvedi, S.K., Artificial intelligence: Revolutionizing mental health in India. *J. Psychiatry*, 21, 4, 287–290, 2018, doi:10.4103/jp.journal_123_18.
19. Egede, L.E. and Walker, R.J., Digital mental health interventions in vulnerable populations: An equity perspective. *Curr. Psychiatry Rep.*, 22, 7, 38, 2020, doi:10.1007/s11920-020-01168-5.
20. Erb, V., Lutz, W., Zimmermann, M., Andersson, G., Digital psychotherapy: AI-powered solutions in clinical practice. *J. Clin. Psychol.*, 79, 2, 300–316, 2023, doi:10.1002/jclp.23478.
21. Eysenbach, G., The role of AI-powered chatbots in mental health crisis intervention. *JMIR Ment. Health*, 8, 6, e29423, 2021, doi:10.2196/29423.
22. Fitzpatrick, K.K., Darcy, A., Vierhile, M., Delivering cognitive behavioral therapy to young adults with symptoms of depression and anxiety using a fully automated conversational agent (Woebot): A randomized controlled trial. *JMIR Ment. Health*, 4, 2, e19, 2017, doi:10.2196/mental.7785.

23. Fusar-Poli, P., Hijazi, Z., Stahl, D., Steyerberg, E.W., The science of prognosis in psychiatry: A review. *JAMA Psychiatry*, 75, 12, 1289–1297, 2018, doi:10.1001/jamapsychiatry.2018.2530.
24. Galatzer-Levy, I.R., Karstoft, K.I., Statnikov, A., Shalev, A.Y., Quantifying the heterogeneity of PTSD using machine learning. *Depress. Anxiety*, 35, 4, 345–355, 2018, doi:10.1002/da.22729.
25. Greer, T.L., Kurian, B.T., Trivedi, M.H., Personalized digital psychiatry: AI-driven interventions for depression. *Neuropsychopharmacology*, 46, 5, 956–964, 2021, doi: 10.1038/s41386-020-00871-3.
26. Haque, A., Milstein, A., Fei-Fei, L., Illuminating mental health disorders through AI-driven insights. *Nat. Med.*, 28, 5, 791–795, 2022, doi: 10.1038/s41591-022-01755-4.
27. Huckvale, K., Venkatesh, S., Christensen, H., Toward clinical digital phenotyping: AI-driven mental health applications. *Trends Cognit. Sci.*, 23, 10, 776–785, 2019, doi: 10.1016/j.tics.2019.06.008.
28. Jorm, A.F., Mental health literacy and the role of AI-driven interventions. *Aust. New Z. J. Psychiatry*, 54, 10, 989–995, 2020, doi: 10.1177/0004867420949452.
29. Kellmeyer, P., Sarró, S., Vijverberg, J., Ethical challenges in AI-driven mental health applications. *Front. Psychiatry*, 10, 846, 2019, doi: 10.3389/fpsyt.2019.00846.
30. Koutsouleris, N., *et al.*, Machine learning-based prediction of psychosis. *Lancet Psychiatry*, 5, 10, 735–746, 2018, doi: 10.1016/S2215-0366(18)30256-7.
31. Kumar, R. and Singh, V., AI-based interventions for mental health: Opportunities and challenges in the Indian context. *Indian J. Psychiatry*, 63, 5, 421–428, 2021, doi: 10.4103/psychiatry.IndianJPsychiatry_123_21.
32. Le Glaz, A., *et al.*, Machine learning and suicide prediction: A systematic review. *J. Affective Disord.*, 281, 24–34, 2021, doi: 10.1016/j.jad.2020.11.057.
33. Luxton, D.D., *Artificial intelligence in behavioral and mental health care*, Academic Press, 2016. doi.org/10.1016/B978-0-12-420248-1.00001-5.
34. Luxton, D.D., AI in clinical psychiatry: A roadmap for future research. *Psychiatr. Serv.*, 73, 1, 12–16, 2022, doi: 10.1176/appi.ps.202100034.
35. Lyon, A.R., Koerner, K., Wong, K., Technology-assisted mental health interventions: Bridging the gap between science and practice. *Clin. Psychol. Rev.*, 78, 101844, 2020, doi: 10.1016/j.cpr.2020.101844.

36. Marsh, A., Dobson, K.S., Pusch, D., AI-driven digital cognitive behavioral therapy: Systematic review and meta-analysis. *Clin. Psychol. Rev.*, 74, 101782, 2019, doi: 10.1016/j.cpr.2019.101782.
37. McGinnis, E., McGinnis, M., Richard, L., AI-powered chatbots and mental health care: Opportunities and challenges, MIT Press, 2022.
38. Muñoz, R.F., *et al.*, Digital mental health interventions for depression prevention. *Annu. Rev. Clin. Psychol.*, 17, 337–367, 2021, doi: 10.1146/annurev-clinpsy-101819-112302.
39. Muralidharan, A. and Rajani, K., Integrating artificial intelligence in mental health care: Prospects and ethical challenges in India. *Indian J. Med. Ethics*, 6, 3, 215–220, 2021, doi: 10.20529/IJME.2021.045.
40. Naslund, J.A., *et al.*, Digital technology for global mental health: Opportunities and challenges. *World Psychiatry*, 18, 2, 135–136, 2019, doi: 10.1002/wps.20628.
41. Niemeijer, A., Deeg, D.J.H., Smits, C., Ethics in AI-driven mental health applications: Protecting user privacy. *Ethics Hum. Res.*, 40, 2, 25–30, 2018, doi: 10.1002/ehr.529.
42. Pantic, I., Digital psychiatry and AI: A systematic review. *Int. J. Psychiatry Clin. Pract.*, 25, 3, 213–221, 2021, doi: 10.1080/13651501.2021.1929385.
43. Patel, V. and Agarwal, S., The role of artificial intelligence in addressing mental health challenges in India. *Lancet Psychiatry*, 7, 12, 1029–1030, 2020, doi: 10.1016/S2215-0366(20)30434-3.
44. Rao, T.S.S. and Menon, V., Artificial intelligence and big data analytics: Implications for mental health in India. *Indian J. Social Psychiatry*, 37, 3, 235–241, 2021, doi: 10.4103/ijsp.ijsp_123_21.
45. Russell, S. and Norvig, P., *Artificial Intelligence: A Modern Approach*, 4th ed., Pearson, 2020.
46. Sarkar, S. and Sood, M., AI-driven mobile applications for mental health: The Indian experience. *J. Technol. Behav. Sci.*, 7, 2, 123–130, 2022, doi: 10.1007/s41347-021-00202-5.
47. Sharma, N. and Gupta, S., Digital psychiatry in India: Leveraging AI for improved mental health outcomes. *Asian J. Psychiatry*, 68, 102983, 2022, doi: 10.1016/j.ajp.2022.102983.
48. Shore, J.H., Yellowlees, P., Caudill, R., Telepsychiatry and E-Mental Health, American Psychiatric Association Publishing, 2018.

49. Thakkar, A., Gupta, A., De Sousa, A., Artificial intelligence in positive mental health: A narrative review. *Front. Digital Health*, 2, 123456, 2024, doi: 10.3389/fdgth.2024.123456.
50. Topol, E., *Deep Medicine: How Artificial Intelligence Can Make Healthcare Human Again*, Basic Books, 2019.
51. Topol, E., *The Deep Learning Revolution in Mental Health Care: AI's Role in Personalized Medicine*, Penguin Books, 2023.
52. Weng, W.H., Chung, W., Wang, X., AI in mental health diagnostics: A comparative analysis. *J. Med. Internet Res.*, 25, e49523, 2023, doi: 10.2196/49523.
53. World Health Organization, AI in Mental Health: Ethical and Regulatory Considerations, WHO Press, 2021, Available: https://www.who.int/publications-detail/ai-in-mental-health.
54. Wysa, AI-powered mental health support, 2024, Available: https://www.wysa.io.
55. Woebot Health, Woebot: Your mental health ally, 2024, Available: https://woebothealth.com.
56. Zhou, X., Zhang, F., Chen, J., Advancing digital psychiatry with explainable AI models. *IEEE Trans. Neural Syst. Rehabil. Eng.*, 30, 1012–1023, 2022, doi: 10.1109/TNSRE.2022.3161123.

2

The Ethics of Digital Psychiatry: Balancing Autonomy, Privacy, and Technological Intervention

Sooraj Kumar Maurya

Zakir Husain Delhi College (Evening), University of Delhi, New Delhi, India

Abstract

The integration of digital tools into psychiatry has transformed the field, offering innovative approaches to diagnosis, treatment, and mental health management. However, this technological shift raises profound ethical questions, particularly concerning autonomy, privacy, and the uses of predictive algorithms. This chapter critically examines these concerns through a philosophical lens, addressing the tensions between technological intervention and core ethical principles in psychiatry. Importantly, patient autonomy, a cornerstone of mental healthcare, is massively challenged by algorithmic decision-making, which risks diminishing individual agency in favor of predictive certainty. The chapter reflects how these issues intersect with the philosophical concept of mental privacy as a fundamental human right. Along with this, it also critiques the normative dimensions of predictive algorithms, which promise enhanced diagnostic precision but may perpetuate biases and reduce mental healthcare to quantifiable metrics. The chapter posits a critical reflection of how to balance technological innovation with ethical practice. It advocates the need for transparency, informed consent, and robust data protection measures to safeguard patient trust and well-being. At the end, the chapter appeals for a holistic approach that integrates technological advances with human-centered care, ensuring that the ethical foundations of psychiatry are not compromised in the pursuit of digital innovation.

***Keywords*:** Digital psychiatry, patient autonomy, mental privacy, predictive algorithms, ethical frameworks

Email: sooraj.au998@gmail.com

Raghavendra M. Devadas, Vani Hiremani, Preethi, Praveen Gujjar, Sapna R. and Manoj Shettar (eds.) Psychiatry and Technology, (29–54) © 2026 Scrivener Publishing LLC

2.1 Introduction

The advancing practice of digital psychiatry is an emerging medical practice of combining mental health services with digital technology platforms. With technological advances, mental health diagnose could be done, and we also could have treatment and monitor services to improve both psychiatric service access and effectiveness [1]. Digital psychiatry is becoming increasingly crucial in current mental health practices because it addresses major problems with treatment accessibility and the mental health labels and the shortage of staff resources. According to the World Health Organization [30], the prevalence of modern mental disorder amounts to more than one in eight people all over the world, but digital psychiatry can offer raised efficiency and helped running services on a broader scale [30]. Key advancements in digital psychiatry underscore its transformative potential. Telepsychiatry, through the use of video conferencing and remote communication/video conferencing features, now provide patients with the opportunity to access care in rural and underserved areas as compared to the past. Mental health is managed through mHealth apps *via* mood trackers and meditation and interactive programs of behavioral therapy exercises [2]. However, both predictive algorithms are an advancement of artificial intelligence (AI), which has two essential functions in making personalized treatments more effective and more effective in diagnostic precision. Yet, wearable devices such as smartwatches and biosensors can actually expand our mental health monitoring capacity to a new level by tracking constant physiological information, detecting real-time conditions.

Recent technological advances have caused significant changes to the practice of mental healthcare in its delivery services and monitoring patient health outcomes. Important ethical problems stand regarding digital psychiatry, which need a careful examination. The principle upon which medical ethics rests fundamentally is that of autonomy, and this principle is tested in this area. On the one hand, algorithm-generated suggestions and app-based treatments influence the choices of patients—a bloodstream potentially from the preservation of free decision-making power [3]. There are additional risks to the postoperative surgical procedures until they have corrected. Asthma patients' lives have been thrown into ÜberMedTech. Still, even those predictive algorithms can risk falling to the power of the bias within the training data that are used to support mental healthcare delivery structures [4]. Ethical technology integration is founded upon the delicate balance of the use of technology through the lens of both human rights protection and dignity preservation. In addressing the urgent healthcare needs, it represents an important developmental step in the current psychiatric treatment.

2.2 Foundations of Digital Psychiatry

With technical development, psychiatry develops with each other to construct a digital practice that went over the conventional normative body-to-body counseling. Modern technologies allowed psychiatrists to build long-term relationships with patients, keeping physical records, primarily pertaining to their assessments conducted at clinics [1]. Although this method was useful when focused situations arose, major difficulties are engaged due to the range for service delivery and the ability it was able to have on operations. Digital tools that came to the forefront during the latter part of the 20th century and first decade of 21st century have revolutionized psychiatry by reducing physical and operational obstacles. With electronic health records making patient data processing easier, healthcare continuity was improved, and interdisciplinary teamwork was enhanced.

The availability of smartphones and the internet provided mental health resources to the masses, thereby making it possible for the mass movements to occur in respect of modern-day mental health accessibility. Major advancements in psychiatric medicine were enabled by new patient care delivery methods *via* technological resources such as telepsychiatry and mobile applications. In the early stages of the COVID-19 pandemic, social distancing rules forced healthcare providers to quickly move to remote mental health services. These advancements comprise a change in the paradigm toward integration of technology in the psychiatric services *via* implementation of interdisciplinary teams formed by clinical experts and technology wizards.

Digital psychiatry consists of the full digital solutions that respond to the need of different clinical subspecialties in the area of diagnosis, treatment, and monitoring patients as well as educational initiatives. A leading telepsychiatry segment is the delivery of psychiatric care per video conferencing applications. Telepsychiatry is researched to have successful results to treat anxiety and depression disorders, as well as remove transportation-associated issues and privacy. Telepsychiatry provides the continuity of psychiatric care in rural areas where such treatment option is scarce and limited. Because mHealth applications function on different platforms and are portable, they are popular. To this end, users can use mobile applications to track moods and get cognitive behavioral therapy lessons, as well as educational information about mental health. Interestingly, the evidence-based applications of Moodpath and Woebot are able to provide their users practical insights as well as therapeutic advice. These tools put the power of monitoring a patient's condition into the patient's hands, as well as detect early warning signs. Today, wearable technologies can be used in psychiatry practice to continuously collect real-time information on sleep patterns and many others such as links up to heart rate variability and physical activities. Preemptive support based on the detection of symptoms for early mental health disorder prior to a diagnosis is based on devices such as smartwatches or fitness trackers as devices to speed up detection.

These AI and machine learning (ML) technologies make a contribution to the development of the capabilities of digital psychiatry. This allows for evaluating huge datasets so as to determine important patterns that you easily cannot notice. Increasingly, personalized psychiatric care is being powered by modern AI tools, such as using advanced system analysis to predict patient outcomes and help doctors to formulate customized treatment strategies, and facilitated through chatbots to provide remote mental health assistance. By processing natural language data through algorithms, depression or schizophrenia indicators can be detected within patient communication records [5]. As AI gets better at implementing precise medicine strategies, it moves toward developing more customized treatments for patients across psychiatry.

In the light of digitized psychiatry, the real limitations of psychiatry medicine are overcome by many advantages. The first advantage of digital tools is that the patients can go to the mental health professional anywhere on the patients' space through their virtual tools. Digital psychiatry is paramount to underserved communities because mental health services are often sparse in remote locations. Its remote servicing model provides digital psychiatry with equitable opportunities for the provision of mental healthcare irrespective of geographical distance barriers [1].

However, digital tools are efficient and effective in psychiatric assessments and hasten the accuracy in evaluating and treating the patients. Automated systems and AI algorithms speed up inspections to the point where bias in treatment decisions minimizes. Proper use of patient data in the ML applications tends to predict better treatment outcome than their conventional clinical counterparts, and as a result, doctors make better choice. Combining objective health indicators that are continuously collected by wearable technology systems such that they fill in the gaps of self-reported information allows for highly precise medical evaluations. Digital psychiatry opens the door to redistributed psychiatric services in which populations that have had no access to proper services have the opportunity to get the attention they need. Digital solutions also scale to benefits for scalable population including the low-income, refugees, and the people with limited mobility. Digital platforms have features that make them relative to various languages and culture to retain their relevance against various consumer demographics [6].

Digital psychiatry is happening as an inevitable change of mental healthcare due to progress in technology, which requires finding solutions to enhance accessibility and efficiency. Telepsychiatry and mHealth applications in sync with wearable devices and AI technologies make it possible to develop precise healthcare approaches for psychiatry that are also more inclusive and scalable. These digital psychiatry practices are rapidly changing, and they must be monitored by ethics to advance toward betterment in mental health clients without the encumbrance of biases in social distribution.

2.3 Autonomy in Digital Psychiatry

In medical ethics, the theory of autonomy is important, which asserts that decisions about healthcare should be made uncoerced by the unwilling individual [7]. For instance, because patients in psychiatry often have very significant vulnerabilities and difficulties in making decisions because of mental health conditions, the importance of autonomy seems even greater in psychiatry [8]. According to Kantian ethics, the rational decision-making is something important enough to be respected as human beings should count as ends and not as means [9]. However, the principle of the continuing existence of the person is violated by digital psychiatry in some ways, and in others, it offers opportunities. Digital tools equip patients with personalized care and insights but also create concerns for maintaining patient control with decision-making and truly assuring informed consent.

2.4 Challenges to Autonomy

2.4.1 Algorithmic Decision-Making

AI and ML algorithms' integration into psychiatry incurs complex challenges to the patient autonomy. However, AI systems tend to deliver on diagnostic accuracy and suggested treatments, automatically reducing patient choice. Such algorithms may conflict with what individual patients prefer or value, and it may be based on population-wide data. Furthermore, many AI systems are understood to be "black box"; i.e., the decision-making process of clinicians and patients is opaque. This lack of transparency has the potential to diminish trust and patient control, as people cannot understand or question how recommendations are determined.

2.4.2 Informed Consent

As medical care moves online with digital platforms, informed consent matures into increasingly complicated terrain. In fact, several digital tools and AI systems now introduce complexities that patients cannot understand, often overwhelming them to the level of doubt about the validity of the consent taken. However, the consent agreements of digital tools are often written in terms that convey a language too technical to adequately discern the data exchange or the algorithms processing of information [3]. In patients who are experiencing acute mental health crisis with impairments in their cognitive abilities, true informed consent becomes even more difficult. It is during such critical periods that patients may not fully understand the risks and benefits of using digital tools, raising ethical concerns regarding the application of these technologies [10].

2.4.3 Digital Literacy Disparities

The capacity for digital literacy to be used by different populations is varying in such a great extent. Due to limited access to technology as well as low levels of digital literacy, many users are faced with barriers when trying out digital psychiatric tools. Different socioeconomic disparities, or different age or educational differences, restrict some groups from getting proper care. For example, the uptake of mobile health applications may be lower among older adults or marginalized groups, limiting their ability to independently manage ongoing mental health. These disparities, if left unchecked, could embed existing mental health inequalities, potentially worsening outcomes for groups who are already most vulnerable [11].

2.5 Potential Solutions

2.5.1 Enhancing Transparency in AI Recommendations

To increase the autonomy of patients, transparency of psychiatric tools driven by AI must be improved. The concept of explainable AI (XAI) is the emergent field of creating algorithms that reveal the knowledge in the algorithm around how a decision was reached [12]. This would not be transparent to patients and would not allow them understand and evaluate the interventions suggested by the AI systems before making informed decisions aligned with their preferences. Furthermore, digital tools have to be communicated in terms that can be understood by patients in terms of advantages, limitations, and potential biases of the digital tool by healthcare providers, to establish trust and autonomy.

2.5.2 Educating Patients about Digital Tools

As it pertains to the patient education, digital psychiatry needs to focus on empowering the patients and increasing their autonomy. There are initiatives that enhance digital literacy to spotlight how digital tools can help patients become aware and familiar with digital tools to make decisions about their healthcare. Given the digital divide and limited time and effectiveness of traditional educational sources, community-based workshops and online educational resources focusing on patients' needs with diverse demographics can help to bridge this gap and facilitate patient engagement [13]. It can also help foster understanding in integrating digital health education into routine clinical interactions with techniques such as the teach-back method to ensure that the patient not only understands the information provided but is able to do so as well [14].

However, digital tools respect and adapt to patients' cultural values, beliefs, and preferences if it is done with cultural competence. Therefore, digital solutions created are collaborative and inclusive and include a base of development teams, healthcare providers, and communities [15]. The enabling of digital health through multiple languages and relevant cultural formats allows healthcare systems to overcome barriers to care, removing barriers to care and allowing all patients to participate in and receive digital psychiatry. The involvement of a diverse range of populations in the testing and development phases of digital tools can also serve to identify biases in the tool, and the tool will be both equitable and effective for all groups. Digital tools in psychiatry hold significant opportunities as well as ethical opportunities to respect patient autonomy. The field of digital psychiatry can address these issues as algorithmic decision-making, informed consent, and digital literacy disparities and, by doing so, protect the autonomy of patients. Empowering patients and protecting their right of self-determination mean promoting transparency in the AI systems, patient education,, and cultural competence with the digital health tools. These efforts can ensure that digital psychiatry keeps evolving in the way that positions patient empowerment and ethically sound practice.

2.6 Privacy Concerns in Digital Psychiatry

Traditionally, mental healthcare values privacy, and this is reflected in the Hippocratic Oath, which states that it is important to protect a patient's information [16]. In psychiatry, in the field where people have to come and let down their guard and disclose things that are very personal and very sensitive, it becomes especially important. Confidentiality assures both patients and clinicians that information is private, which encourages trust between the two groups and allows them easy communication as well as accurate diagnosis [8]. At the same time, the relationship between privacy and the outcome of treatment is established; patients who do not trust the unauthorized disclosure of their data may withhold information important for optimum care [17]. These dynamics highlight the ethical obligations of both mental health professionals and online psychiatry platforms themselves to protect patients' privacy.

Digital psychiatry tools and techniques, such as mobile apps and telehealth platforms, have increased data collection in mental healthcare.

Although these tools provide unprecedented opportunity for more personalized treatment, they also create significant risk to patient privacy. This problem is evident by high-profile data breaches that include a 2020 breach of mental health app that leaked the personal information of thousands of users including their diagnoses and therapy notes. These incidents then as well impact both the legal and psychological consequences.

Mental privacy is defined beyond traditional confidentiality concerns as the ability to protect people's thoughts, emotions, and mental states while they are private. The combination of advances in neurotechnology and AI-driven analysis has generated worries about a possible breach of mental privacy. One such example could be that tools used to analyze facial expressions or speech patterns to infer emotional states could be used for surveillance or manipulation without people's knowledge [18]. It is seen that existing frameworks—particularly privacy by design such as the General Data Protection Regulation (GDPR)—will be addressing data protection itself, but may not completely address the emerging technologies that are further exploring the mind such as protocols that probe mental states. This means there is a need for updated regulations that explicitly protect mental privacy.

The commercialization of health data is another significant threat to privacy in digital psychiatry. A large number of digital health platforms make money by selling patient data to third-party advertisers or researchers. Although practices such as these may encourage innovation, they also confront ethical concerns regarding exploiting vulnerable populations for profit [19]. In most cases, patients do not know how their data are used, as data are encrypted in obscure terms of service agreements. This lack of transparency questions the lack of informed consent and poses normative moot questions surrounding the commodification of health information [20]. This is why robust data protection laws are essential, to address privacy concerns. These frameworks serve as foundation for protecting patient information; examples of such frameworks are the European Union's GDPR and the US Health Insurance Portability and Accountability Act.

These regulations include explicit consent for the use of collected data, defined right of portability of data, and strict regulations for breaches. Nevertheless, the global aspect of digital psychiatry necessitates the development of harmonized international standards in this matter, for the sake of cross-border data flows and major privacy concerns in mental healthcare. This necessitates that policymakers work together to create unified rules that will foster desirable protection for patient data. However, protecting privacy depends heavily on technological solutions. Encryption, such as end-to-end encryption, prevents unauthorized access to data, preserving its integrity during the transmission and storage. Moreover, access control mechanisms such as multifactor authentication and role-based access restrict the access of data to authorized personnel. Therefore, there are also anonymization techniques that can protect patient identities while still allowing aggregated data to be used for research and analysis [21]. Therefore, such privacy safeguards should be inherently built into the design of digital psychiatry platforms.

The regulatory landscape for digital psychiatry has a key role for policymakers. They have to make laws and enforce them and even have to change the rules and regulations to fit into the new technological advancements. For instance, AI for the ethical use in mental healthcare should find ways to deal with issues of bias, transparency, and accountability [22]. Similarly, it is important that public awareness campaigns help patients as far as possible know their rights and the importance of privacy. Through these education efforts, we give users the power to learn how their data are collected, stored, and used to make being educated the most powerful protest of all: choosing to protect your privacy yourself.

Digital psychiatry, by definition, is a multifaceted and sociotechnical phenomenon with much happening both within and outside of the basic technology that emerges from composite components, leading to the involvement of ethics, technology, and policy. The benefits of digital tools for mental healthcare mean they have the potential improve care, but they must not breach patient privacy. It will be necessary for clinicians, technologists, and policymakers to work in conjunction to address the threats such as data breaches, violations of mental privacy, and the commercialization of health data. Through strengthened data protection laws, use of technical safeguards, and transparency, the discipline of digital psychiatry can adhere to ethical principles that properly constitute appropriate mental healthcare.

2.7 Ethical Dimensions of Predictive Algorithms

Psychiatric care has undergone a fundamental and important shift through predictive algorithms that both increase diagnostic precision while generating personalized treatment strategies. The algorithms' capability to examine vast data enables them to detect elusive patterns that human clinicians miss, thus enhancing diagnostic quality. Through ML approaches, researchers show excellent performance in spotting initial psychiatric warning symptoms for depression and schizophrenia, hence achieving rapid intervention and controlling disorder progression. The advanced precision capabilities allow health professionals to design care plans specifically for each patient based on unique biological makeups and environmental circumstances. The combination of these methods results in more effective treatments that produce fewer side effects, thereby generating superior treatment outcomes [23].

The ethical problems connected to predictive algorithms present many different complexities and numerous difficulties. The main ethical dilemma in algorithmic decision systems arises from bias in their algorithms. Algorithms developed using historical data are affected by the biases that exist within those databases because they operate based on historical data. The lack of minority groups in mental health data leads to faulty algorithm performance especially for these populations, which positions new healthcare inequalities. The collection of biased information that results in overidentifying or underidentifying specific population groups causes these inequalities to intensify. The biases that affect data also manifest in the development process of algorithms. The inadequate treatment of these biases could trigger discriminatory results, which diminish predictive technology acceptability along with deepening ethical problems within psychiatric practice [24]. One major ethical problem arises when predictive algorithms simplify mental health conditions by using reductionist models. These algorithms simplify mental health conditions when they rely solely on measurable metrics such as symptom counts or biological indicators. The rigid reductionist perspective overlooks personal patient experiences and ignores social along with cultural influences that affect mental health [28]. The excessive dependence on algorithms in psychiatric practice threatens to convert comprehensive human-centered care into mechanical protocols that risks reducing human connection between mental health practitioners and patients.

The utilization of black-box algorithms that operate with unexplained decision-making logic makes the ethical environment more complex. The systems lacking interpretability produce decision outcomes, which remain unexplained with no notions about their computational reasoning. The absence of transparency enables patients together with clinicians to form mistrust of algorithmic choices, thus preventing comprehensive understanding or detection of algorithmic decision validity. The inability to view inside these systems prevents accountability because errors or biases in algorithms become impossible to identify or repair. Both trust and patient care decisions depend heavily on maintaining transparent systems that enable patients to understand their healthcare process fully. The practice of informed consent could become compromised when healthcare professionals lack full understanding of algorithm operations, which leads to substantial ethical issues in deploying these systems.

The implementation of predictive algorithms has delivered notable successes within psychiatric fields despite significant obstacles. The analysis of text communications by Crisis Text Line ML models has helped identify persons at suicide risk, which enables targeted interventions to save lives through enhanced prioritization of high-risk individuals [25]. By using predictive algorithms, researchers are able to track social media platforms for detecting mental health concerns, allowing them to reach out to affected individuals in advance. The approaches mentioned demonstrate AI's capability to shift public health response capabilities as well as improve mental healthcare access. The use of predictive algorithms has led to various instances of failure that demonstrate the dangerous ethical vulnerabilities in this technology. The public learned about a healthcare algorithm that distributed fewer resources to Black patients through flawed training data, which demonstrates the essential requirement of bias control in algorithm development [4]. The negative effects of predictive algorithm failures intensify within psychiatry because mental health conditions carry extra social discrimination and vulnerability risks. The widespread implementation of predictive algorithms necessitates strict validation procedures and testing approaches to prevent their failures.

Psychiatry should follow several guidelines to achieve responsible algorithm deployment for predictive analytics. The use of diverse representative datasets should serve as a fundamental requirement when training algorithms. Integrating data from minority populations into these systems helps achieve better generalization and fairness, which minimizes healthcare disparities [26]. Henceforth, XAI needs to evolve as a main requirement to enhance the visibility of algorithmic decisions. XAI systems make algorithmic decision processes understandable, which results in enhanced trustworthiness and greater accountability, thus enabling patients and clinicians to understand recommendation rationale [12]. The regular evaluation of predictive algorithms remains vital for both achieving bias-free outcomes together with ethical standards. The ongoing evaluation through audits enables identification of biases and improves performance while maintaining public trust. The auditorial process must consist of medical ethicists together with clinicians and technologists because predictive systems incorporate intricate ethical and technical complexities. The government must create laws to enforce both complete visibility of AI systems and scheduled auditing processes, which should apply specifically to psychiatry applications and others of equal importance.

The future of psychiatric care appears promising with predictive algorithms, which help improve diagnostic outcomes and create customized treatment plans. The effective ethical utilization of predictive algorithms depends on handling issues related to bias along with reductionist and transparent system implementation. The ethical use of predictive algorithms in psychiatric care depends on stakeholder implementation of diverse datasets alongside XAI development and routine auditing procedures. The integration of ethical innovation stands as a vital requirement for attaining the maximum transformative advantages of these emerging technologies.

2.8 Ethical Frameworks for Digital Psychiatry

2.8.1 Deontological Ethics

The moral decision-making model developed by Immanuel Kant through deontological ethics focuses on applying ethical principles and moral duties. The digital psychiatric context requires three essential ethical principles of confidentiality alongside informed consent and patient welfare priority as fundamental decision-making tools [7]. These fundamental principles create a basis for patient–provider trust because they ensure digital interventions maintain patient dignity and autonomy. Digital psychiatry requires physicians to maintain strict confidentiality because the wide data exchange across platforms substantially increases privacy risks. Failure to maintain patient confidentiality damages both ethical guidelines and destroys the necessary trust required to fully engage patients in healthcare treatment [8]. The deontological obligation requires healthcare practitioners to place patient health first by implementing digital tools that serve treatment objectives instead of organizational goals.

2.8.2 Utilitarian Ethics

Utilitarian ethics according to Bentham and Mill presents a consequence-based ethical theory that aims to create the most good and avoid the most damage [27]. Through this ethical framework, digital psychiatry develops methods to assess new technological tools by evaluating their effectiveness in enhancing mental health benefits for broad patient groups. Digital diagnostic systems supported by AI as well as mobile health applications bring multiple advantages because they allow greater access to healthcare services and help identify mental health illnesses early while providing customized treatment options. The assessment required by utilitarian ethics to determine security threats, biases, and diminished human contact in psychiatric care stands as essential [22]. Digital psychiatry operations need to establish a careful equilibrium between their instrument-wide benefits and their associated risks to provide broad population benefits without diminishing therapeutic quality.

2.8.3 Virtue Ethics

Aristotle's philosophical basis of virtue ethics directs healthcare professionals to develop specific virtues in their character rather than emphasizing rule following or consequence-based approaches. Digital psychiatry has to implement the fundamental ethical virtues of empathy and integrity along with practical judgment to maintain proper ethical conduct. The treatment nature of digital psychiatry makes empathy essential because patients often face feelings of isolation through their remote sessions. Through digital means, healthcare providers should exhibit compassion because it preserves the therapeutic bond between doctors and patients [28]. Digital healthcare practitioners need to utilize their practical knowledge by examining the advantages of AI identification systems against essential clinical confirmation. It remains vital for providers to maintain professional integrity to stop technological and financial rewards from overriding basic moral concepts that protect patient welfare. The embodiment of these ethical virtues enables practitioners to handle digital psychiatric challenges while maintaining technology benefits that align with fundamental moral values.

Digital psychiatric practice requires an ethics framework with multiple components that harmonizes the essential principles of deontological ethics with those of utilitarianism and virtue ethics.

Digital mental healthcare requires multiple ethical frameworks because a single theory alone cannot address all the emerging issues [7]. Deontological ethics protects patient privacy by emphasizing the importance of consent. Utilitarianism, on the other hand, evaluates the overall benefits of tools or actions for society. Virtue ethics focuses on providing care with compassion and wisdom. The combined framework supports healthcare providers to defend their patients' self-determination and investigate social effects while maintaining compassionate and ethical behavior. To establish ethical frameworks in digital psychiatry, cooperation between ethicists alongside technologists as well as clinicians and policymakers should develop guidelines that harmonize ethical principles alongside digital age–specific issues [22].

Digital psychiatry enables revolutionary mental health advancements yet creates substantial dilemmas for ethical considerations. The integration of deontology together with utilitarianism and virtue ethics systems enables practitioners to handle digital psychiatric treatment complexities while defending patient autonomy and privacy protection and clinical well-being. The combination of these ethical frameworks establishes an entire system for making ethical decisions in digital psychiatry allowing healthcare professionals to create policies that both respect patient rights and deliver social value. Moreover, the normative principles need integration with digital psychiatry practice to harness technological progress while maintaining human dignity and ensuring equitable and desirable access to care.

2.9 Balancing Innovation with Human-Centered Care

2.9.1 The Need for Balance

Digital technologies integrated in psychiatry practice provide essential benefits, which include better diagnostic precision and tailored treatment designs. The advancement of digital technology needs to preserve essential human qualities central to psychiatric care. Using technology as a higher priority than human contact produces negative effects such as decreased personalized care and diminishing patient–practitioner trust [28].

Psychiatric care requires the therapeutic alliance among patients and clinicians because it depends on empathy combined with trust and open communication according. Too heavy reliance on digital tools weakens their symbiotic relationship with humans because it diminishes personal meetings and shifts essential medical responsibilities toward algorithmic systems. AI systems and chatbots solve immediate problems, but they fall short when it comes to acknowledging genuine patient emotions because they do not possess real empathy abilities. The adoption of digital psychiatry tools raises concerns because they could choose to serve scalability and operational efficiency instead of individual care needs. The fast pace of technological innovation and adaptation often produces a situation where ethical considerations get pushed aside because it leads to problems including data misuse and algorithmic bias alongside limited access to services among marginalized communities [22]. The successful combination of innovative developments and compassionate patient care practices ensures therapy technology operates as a supportive system rather than eliminating humanity from psychiatry practice.

2.9.2 Transparent Communication with Patients

Human-centered care needs transparent communication as its fundamental element when applied to digital psychiatry. The psychiatric treatment outcome depends on patients receiving comprehensive information about digital tools in their care including their advantages and drawbacks along with possible threats [7]. As part of clear communication, practitioners should detail security and privacy aspects regarding patient data while assuring patients about the protection of sensitive information.

2.9.3 Strengthening Informed Consent Processes

The ethical principle known as informed consent provides patients with the freedom to decide whether they want to use digital tools for their healthcare needs. Digital technology implementation requires patient access to comprehensive details about system operation and intended purposes and associated risks [10]. Professional healthcare providers need to use nontechnical language to clearly explain healthcare concepts and digital tool implications to patients so they can fully understand their consequences. The teach-back method serves as a helpful assessment tool because patients need to retell the information they received, which helps verify their understanding [14]. The process of informed consent should continue as patients receive repeated opportunities to modify their decisions when they encounter new information or technological advancements.

2.9.4 Regular Evaluation of Digital Tools for Ethical Alignment

The evaluation process of psychiatric digital tools needs to happen consistently to verify their ethical compliance and their focus on patient-centered approaches. The evaluation process needs to assess digital tools regarding their effectiveness in addition to fairness as well as their impact on patient well-being [22]. Auditing procedures help detect algorithmic biases, which disproportionately impact particular demographic collections; hence, developers can find solutions in advance. The evaluation of ethical concerns needs to investigate the associated implications of digital tools, which can lead to persistent barriers blocking access to medical care for people in need. The evaluation process benefits from stakeholder diversity when ethicists join clinicians and patients to review applications through a collaborative approach, which promotes accountability [29]. Evaluation data from patients should be included to verify that digital equipment fulfills their requirements while preserving psychiatric care's human-centered model.

The integration of sophisticated technology with traditional mental healthcare must be studied through a deliberate method that protects human values. Technological advancements have the ability to boost mental health results, yet their implementation should never undermine the therapeutic relationship or diminish trust between patients and healthcare providers. The integration of digital tools requires medical practitioners to maintain open communication while enhancing patient consent procedures and conducting periodic evaluations of their digital systems to strike this equilibrium. The advancement of digital psychiatry depends on uniting innovative techniques with respect for human emotions and ethical principles.

2.10 Recommendations for Ethical Digital Psychiatry

To address the normative complexities that are intrinsically part of digital psychiatry requires a comprehensive regulatory framework. The patient privacy, data security, and equitable access to digital mental health tool must be priorities in policy. International standards such as the GDPR provide a foundation from which to ensure person's personal health and care data are protected by explicit consent and data minimization. Such frameworks should be tailored to the particular challenges of digital psychiatry, emphasizing transparency in the algorithmic decision-making process, and appropriate response in terms of accountability and responsibility of those who provide those platforms.

In addition, digital mental health resources have to be made accessible to everyone directly through the regulations. It entails promoting the creation of culturally responsive technologies or the limited distribution of digital psychiatry technological solutions to underserved populations to avoid exploitation and achieve equity [22]. In order to lower barriers to care for marginalized groups, public funding initiatives should help provide for the creation of open-access platforms that prioritize inclusivity and affordability. It is vital for digital psychiatry that clinicians maintain the ethical standards.

Clear, transparent communication around benefits, risks, and limitations of digital tools is required for a patient-centered approach. Therefore, informed consent in the case of implementation of digital technologies requires identifying and addressing the possible concerns and provides explanations of how digital technologies work, for example [10]. It is essential to provide professional development for ongoing support of new skills required to undertake digital psychiatry in the field of ethics. There should be training programs that include data ethics, alien transparency, and biases in the AI system [7]. Clinicians also need to practice regular self-reflection to establish that the use of the technology is in keeping with the core principles of the use of empathy, integrity, and respect for patient autonomy. There are existing gaps in the ethical understanding of digital psychiatry that required further research. An important area for research is in the development of XAI systems, which can derive and explain the reasoning behind their decisions [12]. In particular, they are essential to having trust and empowering both clinicians and patients to know what decisions they should make based on the logic of AI intervention.

Furthermore, digital psychiatry research should be carried out on the effects of the therapeutic alliance and mental health outcomes in the long term. This is important to studies exploring the sociocultural impacts of digital tools and their potential to exacerbate or ameliorate health disparities [28]. The incremental ethical evolution of digital psychiatry can be informed by collaborative research efforts that involve ethicists, technologists, and clinicians, which can generate nuanced insights. Ethical digital psychiatry is to be multifaceted, entailing policy development, practitioner guidelines, and research initiatives aimed at understanding and developing the best methods of providing these services. The field has significant opportunity to advance while striving to prioritize patient rights and promote equitable care for all, although by implementing comprehensive regulatory frameworks, strengthening the basis of ethical clinical practices, and addressing knowledge gaps, this can be achieved.

2.11 Conclusion

Digital tools implemented at a fast pace in psychiatry create transformative opportunities alongside substantial ethical dilemmas. The implementation of digital psychiatry requires a well-balanced strategy because it faces major concerns regarding patient autonomy as well as privacy protections and algorithm ethics. To protect autonomy, healthcare providers must enable patients to hold their decisions with importance, even when algorithms recommend actions or digital interventions are used [8]. The requirements for protecting privacy emerge as critical through data safety needs, and ethical violations connected to mental privacy breaches therefore require advanced legal safeguards along with technological measures and procedural protections. The implementation of predictive algorithms for diagnostic purposes and personalized medicine generates essential concerns regarding model bias along with transparency and accountability standards. Digital psychiatry needs ethical considerations such as fundamental principles throughout the development together with implementation stage. Embedded principles of fairness along with empathy and respect throughout technological innovations will help stakeholders create mental health technology that matches basic mental healthcare standards. These ethical principles have a practical significance because they generate trust through patient care enhancements and reduce possible negative effects. These problems need extensive cooperation between multiple different groups. The care profession needs to defend patient-focused treatments with updated knowledge about digital tools' ethical effects on care delivery. The formation of detailed policies by policymakers should cover data management procedures and requirements for transparent algorithms along with rules on equitable platform access. Technologists must develop easily understandable and inclusive technology systems that put user welfare first [12]. Several professional groups find success in creating a complete system that upholds digital psychiatry's ethical standards when they operate together. The objective for future development must involve enhancing traditional care before substituting it with advanced technology instead of seeking direct interchange between human and machine systems. Psychiatric tools should reinforce interpersonal capabilities instead of replacing the person-to-person qualities essential for quality psychiatric treatment. The realization of this vision depends on sustained ethical examination together with strict assessment along with an organizational commitment to patient welfare. Through this citizen-centric method, digital psychiatry reaches its goal and preserves human dignity within patient care.

AI disclosure statement: The author acknowledges the use of AI-based tools for minor language editing or grammatical correction. However, all intellectual contributions, analyses, and conclusions presented in this chapter are entirely the author's own.

References

1. Torous, J. and Roberts, L.W., Needed innovation in digital health and smartphone applications for mental health: Transparency and trust. *JAMA Psychiatry*, *74*, 5, 437–438, 2017, https://doi.org/10.1001/jamapsychiatry.2017.0262.
2. Mohr, D.C., Burns, M.N., Schueller, S.M., Clarke, G., Klinkman, M., Behavioral intervention technologies: Evidence review and recommendations for future research in mental health. *Gen. Hosp. Psychiatry*, 35, 4, 332–338, 2013, https://doi.org/10.1016/j.genhosppsych.2013.03.008.
3. Mittelstadt, B.D., Allo, P., Taddeo, M., Wachter, S., Floridi, L., The ethics of algorithms: Mapping the debate. *Big Data Soc.*, 3, 2, 1–21, 2016, https://doi.org/10.1177/2053951716679679.
4. Obermeyer, Z., Powers, B., Vogeli, C., Mullainathan, S., Dissecting racial bias in an algorithm used to manage the health of populations. *Science*, 366, 6464, 447–453, 2019, https://doi.org/10.1126/science.aax2342.
5. Lake, J. and Kleinman, M., Artificial intelligence and the future of psychiatry: Insights from machine learning and natural language processing. *Curr. Psychiatry Rep.*, 23, 8, 45, 2020.

6. Insel, T.R., Digital phenotyping: Technology for a new science of behavior. *JAMA*, 318, 13, 1215–1216, 2017.
7. Beauchamp, T.L. and Childress, J.F., *Principles of Biomedical Ethics*, Oxford University Press, New York, NY, USA, 2019.
8. Appelbaum, P.S., Assessment of patients' competence to consent to treatment. *N. Engl. J. Med.*, 357, 18, 1834–1840, 2007.
9. Kant, I., *Groundwork of the Metaphysics of Morals*, M. Gregor (Ed. & Trans.), Cambridge University Press, Cambridge, United Kingdom (UK), 1997, (Original work published 1785).
10. Kim, S.Y., Caine, E.D., Currier, G.W., Leibovici, A., Ryan, J.M., Assessing the competence of persons with Alzheimer's disease in providing informed consent for participation in research. *Am. J. Psychiatry, 158*, 5, 712–717, 2001, https://doi.org/10.1176/appi.ajp.158.5.712.
11. Choi, N.G. and DiNitto, D.M., Internet use among older adults: Association with health needs, psychological capital, and social capital. *J. Med. Internet Res.*, 15, 5, e97, 2013.
12. Gunning, D., Stefik, M., Choi, J., Miller, T., Stumpf, S., Yang, G.Z., XAI—Explainable artificial intelligence. *Sci. Rob.*, 4, 37, eaay7120, 2019.
13. Norman, C.D. and Skinner, H.A., eHealth literacy: Essential skills for consumer health in a networked world. *J. Med. Internet Res.*, 8, 2, e9, 2006.
14. Ha Dinh, T.T., Bonner, A., Clark, R., Ramsbotham, J., Hines, S., The effectiveness of the teach-back method on adherence and self-management in health education for people with chronic disease: A systematic review. *JBI Database Syst. Rev. Implementation Rep.*, 14, 1, 210–247, 2016.
15. Betancourt, J.R., Green, A.R., Carrillo, J.E., Ananeh-Firempong, O., Defining cultural competence: A practical framework for addressing racial/ethnic disparities in health and health care. *Public Health Rep.*, 118, 4, 293–302, 2003.
16. Jotterand, F., The Hippocratic oath and contemporary medicine: dialectic between past ideals and present reality? *J. Med. Philos., 30*, 1, 107–128, 2005, https://doi.org/10.1080/03605310590907084.

17. Henderson, C., Evans-Lacko, S., Flach, C., Thornicroft, G., Responses to mental health stigma questions: The importance of social desirability and data collection method. *Can. J. Psychiatry*, *57*, 3, 152–160, 2012, https://doi.org/10.1177/070674371205700304.
18. Ienca, M. and Andorno, R., Towards new human rights in the age of neuroscience and neurotechnology. *Life Sci. Soc. Policy*, 13, 1, 1–27, 2017.
19. Lupton, D., The commodification of patient opinion: The digital patient experience economy in the age of big data. *Sociol. Health Illn.*, 36, 6, 856–869, 2014.
20. Hoffman, S. and Podgurski, A., The use and misuse of biomedical data: Is bigger really better? *Am. J. Law Med.*, *39*, 4, 497–538, 2013, https://doi.org/10.1177/009885881303900401.
21. Ohm, P., Broken promises of privacy: Responding to the surprising failure of anonymization. *UCLA Law Rev.*, 57, 6, 1701–1777, 2010.
22. Floridi, L., Cowls, J., Beltrametti, M., Chatila, R., Chazerand, P., Dignum, V., Schafer, B., AI4People—An ethical framework for a good AI society: Opportunities, risks, principles, and recommendations. *Mines Mach.*, 28, 4, 689–707, 2018.
23. Chekroud, A.M., Bondar, J., Delgadillo, J., Doherty, G., Wasil, A., Fokkema, M., Cohen, Z., Belgrave, D., DeRubeis, R., Iniesta, R., Dwyer, D., Choi, K., The promise of machine learning in predicting treatment outcomes in psychiatry. *World Psychiatry*, *20*, 2, 154–170, 2021, https://doi.org/10.1002/wps.20882.
24. Mehrabi, N., Morstatter, F., Saxena, N., Lerman, K., Galstyan, A., A survey on bias and fairness in machine learning. *ACM Comput. Surv.*, 54, 6, 1–35, 2021.
25. Miner, A.S., Milstein, A., Schueller, S., Smartphone-based conversational agents and responses to questions about mental health, interpersonal violence, and physical health. *JAMA Intern. Med.*, 176, 5, 622–623, 2016.
26. Chen, I.Y., Johansson, F.D., Sontag, D., Why is my classifier discriminatory? Towards automatic removal of bias. *Advances in Neural Information Processing Systems*, vol. 33, pp. 240–253, 2018.
27. Mill, J.S., *Utilitarianism*, Parker, Son, and Bourn, West Strand, 1863.

28. Holmes, E.A., Ghaderi, A., Harmer, C.J., Ramchandani, P.G., Cuijpers, P., Morrison, A.P., Craske, M.G., The Lancet Psychiatry Commission: Future directions for psychological science. *Lancet Psychiatry*, 5, 3, 237–286, 2018.
29. Binns, R., Fairness in machine learning: Lessons from political philosophy. *Proceedings of the 2018 Conference on Fairness, Accountability, and Transparency*, pp. 149–159, 2018.
30. World Health Organization. *World mental health report: Transforming mental health for all.* World Health Organization, Geneva, 2022.

3

Big Data Analytics and Predictive Analytics in Psychiatry: Transforming Mental Healthcare

Gujanatti Rudrappa[1]*, Sushant Jadhav[1], Arun Tigadi[1] and Sachin Urabinahatti[2]

[1]Department of Electronics and Communication, KLE Technological University, Dr. M S Sheshgiri Campus, Belagavi, India
[2]Department of Artificial Intelligence and Machine Learning, BMS Institute of Technology and Management, Bangalore, India

Abstract

The field of psychiatry has experienced a significant transformation due to the rapid advancement of predictive modeling and big data analytics. Traditional psychiatric therapy relied on subjective clinical observations and patients' self-reported symptoms, leading to late diagnosis and treatment experiments. However, big data technology has revolutionized psychiatry by making treatment more accurate, efficient, and scalable using big databases. Predictive analysis has revealed potential manifestations that can be beneficial, and various data sources such as social media activity, genetic data, neuroimaging scans, and electronic health records are analyzed to obtain practical findings. The advent of data science and genomics has enabled scientists and doctors to predict clinical outcomes and tailor treatments with precision. Machine learning and artificial intelligence are used to provide data-driven insights, enabling patients to be nudged toward better survival with the right treatment plan.

The chapter explores the approaches these technologies adopt to tackle mental diseases, focusing on applications such as tailored therapies, relapse prediction, and suicide risk assessment. It also addresses ethical issues, algorithmic biases, and data integration difficulties. The future directions include augmented psychiatry and global mental health endeavors, where big data and predictive analytics can change mental illness treatment.

**Corresponding author*: rudraguj@gmail.com

Raghavendra M. Devadas, Vani Hiremani, Preethi, Praveen Gujjar, Sapna R. and Manoj Shettar (eds.) Psychiatry and Technology, (55–90) © 2026 Scrivener Publishing LLC

***Keywords*:** Psychiatry, predictive modeling, big data analytics, machine learning (ML), artificial intelligence (AI), data science, genomics

3.1 Introduction

In the past, the practice of psychiatry, a medical field that studies mental health and behavioral issues, has generally had to rely on personal interpretations and clinical findings as the major components of diagnosis and therapy. Nevertheless, the novel areas of big data analytics and predictive modeling can transform this field by helping caregivers offer more evidence-based and objective services. Big data, for example, are a vast and complex dataset produced by different sources. Channels such as electronic health records (EHRs), neuroimaging, genomics, personal wearable devices, and social media platforms are examples of these sources. These data can unveil patterns that have never been seen before, discover risk factors, and predict the outcome, providing doctors with more information on their patients' diagnosis and treatment of illness.

A discipline of big data analytics that goes by the name of predictive analytics applies unique algorithms, such as machine learning (ML) and artificial intelligence (AI), to foresee treatment outcomes and tailor interventions to specific patient needs at an individual level. Predictive analytics is a valuable tool in the treatment process, for example, by assisting in the diagnosis, getting an early intervention, and treatment response variability in the psychiatry sector, which means that diseases such as depression, anxiety, schizophrenia, and bipolar disorder (BPD) often occur in different forms. For example, sequences of depression, environmental influences, genetic mutations, and psychiatric history, which become manifest after long-time adaptations, can be viewed. The AI that has been trained with big sets of data can already detect mental health problems and forecast the probability of relapse, providing doctors with manifestly implemented tools for preventive care [1, 2].

The great potential of psychiatry concerning the use of large quantities of data and predictive analytics is due to the diversity of data sources that can be used for these purposes [3]. An anatomic as well as functional disorder of the brain can be revealed through neuroimaging, whereas genomic investigations will show disorders of a genetic nature [4]. The following is a more detailed analysis of digital phenotyping, which will help you better understand the differences and similarities between these two analyses. The data collected through sensors and devices of smartphones, which is later transformed into digital phenotyping, can be used to monitor behavior [5]. The patient's condition and, consequently, the physician's decisions are highly affected by these data. Precision psychiatry can be practiced with a combination of several data streams, such as genomic data, environmental data, wearable biosensors data, etc. One of the primary questions raised by the authors in this chapter is the potentiality of big data and predictive analytics that can be utilized in the field of psychiatry. They have thoroughly analyzed the various uses, such as early diagnosis of diseases, suicide prevention, and personalized medicine, and addressed the moral and practical concerns linked to the application of these instruments in the clinical sector. Additionally, the study explores the most important sources and technical breakthroughs underlying this transformation. The primary intent of the chapter is to present a whole picture of how decision-making in the area of mental health is affected by the new technology such as the real-life examples and future treatments.

3.2 Data Sources in Psychiatry

It is predicted that the area of psychiatry will gain the most from the use of big data due to the fact that the generated data are of different types, coming from digitalization, behavior, clinical, and biological sources. Combining data from different sources will result in more accurate predictive models for diagnosis, therapy, and prognosis. Thus, the aforementioned limitations could be solved by delving deeper into the data, combining different approaches and data from various sources, and not relying on a single approach or source. This allows us to get a broader view and better acquainted with mental health issues. The objective of the section is to discuss the top sources of psychiatric data.

3.2.1 Electronic Health Records

EHRs are electronic databases that contain both unstructured and structured information about the patients' health [6]. Structured data are composed of items such as diagnoses, medication records, and laboratory outcomes. Unstructured data could be said to relate to clinical records and resources. EHRs are beneficial to psychiatry primarily because it enables the doctors to view the progress of their patients and thus see trends in the data of their patients, track the efficiency of their treatments, and predict results by the analysis of past data. Among the most challenging ones are the issues of data interoperability between systems and patient privacy.

Example: One use of EHRs is in predicting incidents of dementia [7].

3.2.2 Neuroimaging Data

Electroencephalography (EEG), positron emission tomography (PET), functional magnetic resonance imaging (fMRI), and magnetic resonance imaging (MRI) are some of the neuroimaging techniques that help us understand the brain's structure and function.

Applications:

- Locating indicators of mental diseases such as BPD or schizophrenia.
- Recognizing how disorders of depression and anxiety impact alterations in connection.

Example: Neuroimaging research has revealed that those suffering from major depressive disorder (MDD) had less connection in the prefrontal brain [8].

3.2.3 Genomic and Proteomic Data

The biological bases of mental health issues can be better understood with the use of genomics and proteomics.

- **Genomics**: Its primary emphasis is on the genetic variants linked to mental illness. Autism spectrum disorder (ASD), BPD, and schizophrenia have all been related to specific genes, according to Genome-Wide Association Studies (GWAS).
- **Proteomics**: It investigates patterns of protein expression to learn about the molecular processes at work in mental diseases.

Example: The Psychiatric Genomics Consortium has effectively identified genetic risk factors for diseases such as schizophrenia and major depression [9].

3.2.4 Wearable Devices and Digital Phenotyping

Cellphones and wearable technology have made it possible to track patients' vital signs and behavioral patterns in real time. This information, often called digital phenotyping, records how active a person is, how much sleep they get, their heart rate, and even their typing or speaking habits. Researchers have utilized Fitbit data to evaluate sleep disruptions experienced by persons suffering from anxiety disorders [10].

Applications:

- Detecting the first symptoms of mental illness
- Keeping an eye on the likelihood of relapse and how consistent medication use is

3.2.5 Social Media and Online Behavior

Social media platforms, blogs, and forums are becoming more and more relevant data sources when it comes to public mental health trends and identifying individual mental health issues. Tweets, postings, and messages can be analyzed using natural language processing (NLP) to detect emotional states or thoughts of suicide. Fatigue or lack of energy was the most common depressive symptom, whereas feelings of worthlessness were the least common, according to the study presented by researchers [11]. Findings from the study indicate that public mental health hotspots that are on the decline could be better addressed with the use of Twitter data [11].

3.2.6 Surveys and Psychometric Instruments

Established questionnaires and psychometric methods are still critical in the field of psychiatry. They consist of scales administered by the clinic personnel; the scales considered are the Hamilton Depression Rating Scale and the Patient Health Questionnaire-9, as well as self-reported questionnaires. The advantages are that they directly assess mood, cognition, and actions. Challenges evolve around self-reports reliability, which can be limited due to their subjectivity and variability.

3.2.7 Environmental and Socioeconomic Data

Factors in the environment, including urbanization, air pollution, and socioeconomic position, significantly impact mental health. Combining psychiatric datasets with geographic information systems and environmental parameters helps us understand these factors better. For instance, according to research by Braithwaite *et al.* [12], mental health issues, including anxiety and depression, are more likely to develop in those who are exposed to more air pollution.

Table 3.1 provides a detailed summary of the various data sources, the challenges imposed while utilizing the psychiatric data sources, and their impact.

Table 3.1 Summary of data sources, the challenges in utilizing psychiatric data sources, and their impact.

Data source	Description	Challenges	Impact
Electronic health records (EHRs)	Longitudinal patient records containing structured and unstructured data	Data inconsistency across systems, missing or incomplete data entries, interoperability challenges.	Reduces data reliability and predictive accuracy.
Neuroimaging data	Imaging techniques such as MRI, fMRI, PET, and EEG to study brain structure and function	High cost and technical expertise required, variability in data quality between imaging centers, complex processing workflows.	Limits scalability and generalizability for population-level analysis.
Genomic and proteomic data	Genetic and protein expression data to identify biomarkers for psychiatric disorders	Expensive and resource, intensive collection processes, ethical concerns regarding genetic privacy, limited availability of representative datasets.	Delays advancements in precision psychiatry and excludes diverse populations.
Wearable devices and digital phenotyping	Continuous behavioral and physiological monitoring through wearables and smartphones	Data reliability is affected by device accuracy and user compliance, privacy concerns related to real-time data collection, integration of heterogeneous streams of data.	Challenges real-time predictive applications and risks breaches of sensitive patient information.

(*Continued*)

Table 3.1 Summary of data sources, the challenges in utilizing psychiatric data sources, and their impact. (*Continued*)

Data source	Description	Challenges	Impact
Social media and online behavior	Textual and behavioral data from social media platforms to infer mental health trends	- Ethical concerns around consent and user anonymity. - Noisy data with high variability - Risk of misclassification due to language and cultural differences.	May produce biased models or incorrect predictions, impacting reliability in clinical settings.
Surveys and psychometric tools	Self-reported data from validated questionnaires and clinician-administered scales	Subjective and prone to bias or misreporting, variability in scoring due to differences in clinical interpretation, limited data collection over time.	Results in incomplete or nonrepresentative datasets affecting predictive model performance.
Environmental and socioeconomic data	Data on factors such as urbanization, pollution, and socioeconomic status impacting mental health	Difficulty in linking environmental metrics to individual psychiatric data, Limited availability of granular, localized data.	Fails to account for environmental contributions to mental health disorders fully.

3.3 Key Technologies in Big Data Analytics in Psychiatry

Big data analytics is making use of sophisticated approaches or technologies, which is represented in Figure 3.1. These technologies process the big data; once processed, it can analyze it and then obtain

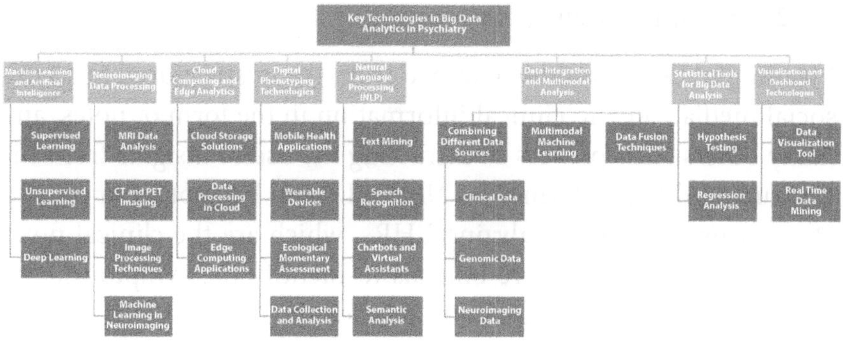

Figure 3.1 Key technologies in big data analytics in psychiatry.

the key insights. Researchers and medical specialists can derive important insights from the data by using the state-of-art methods and make predictions accordingly. Brief details of the key technologies utilized in psychiatric big data analytics are presented above.

3.3.1 ML and AI

ML and AI have become an essential component in the study of psychiatric big data. The algorithms that leverage ML and AI features learn the pattern from the data (primary or secondary) during the training phase and leverage the learning for making the predictions. These algorithms are basically categorized as supervised algorithms and unsupervised algorithms.

In supervised algorithms, the algorithms need to be trained in the data that have been labeled. For instance, support vector machines (SVMs) and random forests were used for prediction of suicidal risk tendency by utilizing the EHR data [13].

In unsupervised algorithms, the algorithms are trained by using the data that are not labeled. For example, algorithms for clustering patient groups by the response to treatment can be obtained by utilizing k-means clustering approach.

Apart from the supervised and unsupervised algorithms, few algorithms use deep learning (DL), which can work with high-dimensional data. For example, convolutional neural networks were utilized for classifying the MRI images to identify Alzheimer disease [14].

3.3.2 Natural Language Processing

Meaningful details can be obtained from the unstructured text, viz., social media content, clinical information in the form of notes, and many others. This process of extracting the useful insights from the unstructured text is termed as NLP. NLP can be applied in psychiatry, for example, for analyzing EHRs, which are the clinical notes recorded by the healthcare officials to identify the symptoms, and then detail out the diagnoses and provide the required medications. For example, disorders in the mood of the patient have been identified by analyzing the patients' written and spoken words by leveraging the NLP-based sentiment analysis [15].

3.3.3 Neuroimaging Data Processing

To understand how the brain of a human functions in case of patients with psychiatric problems, identifying the biomarkers becomes vital task. The biomarker identification requires using methods such as neuroimage data processing. For example, graph theory was used for analyzing the brains of patients with schizophrenia. Now, much more advanced approaches are leveraging the benefits of using ML algorithms for classification of neuroimages to diagnose the conditions such as autism or MDD. For instance, for classifying the BPD in mental health patients, SVMs were used for fMRI images [16].

3.3.4 Data Integration and Multimodal Analysis

Psychiatric big data often involve diverse data types, including genetic, behavioral, and environmental data. Integrating these datasets requires robust platforms and methodologies.

- **Multimodal data integration tools**: TensorFlow and PyTorch are tools that allow for the integration of heterogeneous datasets to gain a complete view.

Example: Neuroimaging data with genetic markers to predict risk for schizophrenia.

- **Big data platforms**: Apache Hadoop and Spark allow for massive storage and parallel processing of large-scale psychiatric datasets.

3.3.5 Cloud Computing and Edge Analytics

Cloud computing will allow psychiatric big data to be stored and analyzed on scalable remote servers, but edge analytics would process the data locally at its source for quicker responses.

- **Cloud platforms**: Amazon Web Services and Google Cloud are most popularly used in storing and analyzing massive datasets such as genomic studies or EHRs.
- **Edge computing**: Worn, and the first process of that relates to handling patient data in real time. By doing so, latency in monitoring certain symptoms or behaviors is thereby reduced.

Example: Monitoring speech patterns with use of smartphones for BPD patients.

3.3.6 Statistical Tools for Big Data Analysis

Statistical tools are essential for the processing and analysis of psychiatric data so as to identify valuable patterns or relationships.

- **Bayesian models**: Useful in doing probabilistic reasoning, that, for example, would predict the likelihood of success at treatment.
- **Regression analysis**: This technique helps to find correlations between variables, such as socioeconomic factors and mental health outcomes.

Example: Cox proportional hazards models are often used in survival analysis to predict relapse.

3.3.7 Digital Phenotyping Technologies

Digital phenotyping is the use of smartphones, wearables, and apps to monitor behavior and physiology continuously.

- **Data collection technologies**: Accelerometers measure movement, and heart rate monitors measure stress responses.

Example: Apps such as Mindstrong use passive data collection to predict depressive episodes.

- **Analysis platforms**: Processed sensor data will be used by MATLAB and R for the development of meaningful features.

3.3.8 Visualization and Dashboard Technologies

Data visualization products aid clinicians as well as investigators to interpret heavy psychiatric data.

- **Visualization tools**: These include the creation of dashboards as intuitively responsive in monitoring progression for patients and also in portraying brain connectivity.

Example: 3D rendering of data related to neuroimaging.

3.4 Predictive Analytics Applications in Psychiatry

Predictive analytics is the technique of using ML, statistical algorithms, and data mining methods to identify the patterns and make a prediction about the future based on past data. The predictive analytics technique revolutionized mental healthcare by allowing earlier diagnosis, treatment customization, and better outcomes for patients. Here are some of the primary applications of predictive analytics in psychiatry.

3.4.1 Early Diagnosis of Mental Health Disorders

Early diagnosis of psychiatric disorders is key to proper treatment and better long-term prognosis. Predictive models take into account diverse datasets that capture subtle patterns prior to the emergence of psychiatric disorders. From an early intervention point of view, disorder progression is stopped. For example:

- ML models trained on EHRs and family history data were able to predict the probability of developing schizophrenia or BPD years before clinical onset [17].
- Smartphone-based digital phenotyping tracks behavioral dynamics to detect early-warning signs of depression [18].

3.4.2 Treatment Response Prediction

Because mental disorders are relatively heterogeneous, psychiatric treatments rely mostly on empirical methods. Predictive analytics resolve this by giving more focused and targeted treatment based on the unique characteristics of that patient, thereby reducing the time to find effective treatment and minimizing patient distress and healthcare costs. For example:

- Genetic data have been used to predict response to antidepressants such as selective serotonin reuptake inhibitors [19].
- Combining demographic, clinical, and neuroimaging data enhances the accuracy of predictions [20].

3.4.3 Suicide Risk Assessment

Predictive analytics has proven to be quite promising in suicide prevention, a very sensitive area. Predictive models identify those who are likely to commit suicide or attempt suicide based on data retrieved from EHRs, social media, and wearable devices, which gives clinicians actionable insights to prioritize at-risk patients for intervention. For example:

- ML algorithms have been designed to predict the chances of suicide attempts from hospital records with a success rate of 90% [13].
- NLP techniques used on social media posts identify suicidal language or expressions of hopelessness [21].

3.4.4 Relapse Prediction

Relapse rates for mental health conditions such as depression and schizophrenia are high due to incomplete recovery or external triggers. Predictive analytics can monitor the ongoing mental health of patients to foresee and prevent relapses. It facilitates preventive interventions that decrease hospitalization rates and enhance life quality. For example, wearable devices monitoring sleep, activity, and heart rate variability detect biomarkers for BPD relapse [22].

3.4.5 Personalized Interventions

Personalized psychiatry involves delivering evidence-based interventions based on unique patient profiles for enhanced outcome responses. Predictive analytics combines genomic, neuroimaging, and behavioral multivariate data to suggest the appropriate personalized therapies, which aligns treatments with patient-specific needs, enhancing therapeutic efficacy. For example, predictive models use fMRI data determine which patients will benefit from cognitive behavioral therapy (CBT) versus pharmacological treatments [23].

3.4.6 Substance Use Disorder Treatment

Predictive analytics helps discover trends in substance use disorders for early intervention and decreased rates of relapse. This informs the creation of specific rehabilitation programs to allow for prevention and decreases the social burden related to substance abuse. For example, analyzing the EHRs and social determinants of health helped predict the potential for opioid addiction among patients who are prescribed opioids [24].

3.4.7 Mental Health Trend Forecasting

At the population level, predictive analytics will be able to predict trends in mental health disorders, which allows policymakers and healthcare providers to know where to place their resources. This improves response to emerging mental health crises. For example, analytics of social media and search engines were used to forecast increases in anxiety and depression during the COVID-19 pandemic [15].

3.4.8 Posttreatment Monitoring

Posttreatment surveillance is critical in maintaining healing and preventing reemergence of the psychopathology. Predictive analytics monitors mental health over time after treatment, which helps to monitor long-term healthcare management and reduce relapses. For example, mobile applications apply ML algorithms that analyze behavioral and interaction patterns between the patient and the machine and alert signs of deterioration during the postpsychotherapy or post–medication treatment period.

3.4.9 Implementation Challenges

Although predictive analytics is very promising, several challenges have to be met to realize maximum utility. These challenges have been presented in Table 3.2.

Table 3.2 Challenges in utilizing the psychiatric data.

Challenge	Description
Data quality	Missing or noisy data can severely compromise the model's accuracy
Bias in algorithms	Models trained on nonrepresentative datasets may lead to biased predictions
Interpretability	Clinicians need explainable models for effective decision-making
Ethical issues	Ensuring patient confidentiality and data security, especially for sensitive psychiatric data

3.5 Predictive Analysis for Psychiatry: Case Studies and Real-World Examples

Several researchers and healthcare officials have provided key insights into various state-of-the-art techniques for predictive analysis in the domain of psychiatry. Many datasets with different features were also established by various researchers. These important case studies and illustrations help to clarify the developments.

3.5.1 Early Diagnosis of Schizophrenia Using Multimodal Data

To identify those at risk of developing schizophrenia, researchers at the Max Planck Institute for Psychiatry developed a prediction model that would integrate clinical, genetic, and neuroimaging data. With an 81% prediction accuracy for the onset of schizophrenia, longitudinal datasets from high-risk individuals were analyzed using ML algorithms [25]. In order for the physicians to postpone or stop the disease's emergence, early detection was followed by the implementation of prophylactic treatments.

3.5.2 Suicide Attempt Prediction with EHRs

To anticipate patient suicide attempts inside a hospital system, Vanderbilt University conducted research using EHRs.

Model for ML: More than 5000 variables were taken into account by the model. These consist of clinical, pharmaceutical, and demographic data. Eighty percent of at-risk individuals were accurately identified by the algorithm before they actually attempted suicide [13]. The approach saved lives by enabling mental health practitioners to concentrate interventions on patients who were in immediate danger.

3.5.3 Digital Phenotyping for Mood Disorders

In Denmark, the MONARCA study concentrated on monitoring bipolar illness patients with smartphones. Sleep, physical activity, and self-reported mood were all recorded by the system. Manic or depressed episodes were correctly recognized by predictive models [22]. Real-time monitoring was made possible by this method, which enhanced patient involvement in their care and relapse prevention.

3.5.4 Personalized Treatment for Depression with Neuroimaging Data

ML model was developed by the researchers at Weill Cornell Medicine for forecasting the results of treatment to patients suffering from MDD [26]. An accuracy of 80% was recorded for classifying the respondents as healthy or unhealthy for CBT.

3.5.5 Suicide Risk Detection through Social Media Analysis

Witters messages were analyzed by using NLP by the Harvard Computational Psychiatry Lab, to identify users with suicidal tendencies. An accuracy of 85% was achieved by the system used. The unstructured texts from Twitter messages served as hint for the system proposed [15]. These techniques have been utilized within the crisis hotlines and other mental health systems to detect personnel who are at risk of suicidal tendency.

3.5.6 Opioid Use Disorder Prediction

The University of Pittsburgh utilized predictive analytics to detect individuals at high risk who could be addicted to opioids. Accuracy of 88% was achieved with the system, which leveraged the ML algorithms for detecting the addiction of a person toward opioid. The ML algorithm utilized the EHRs along with the socioeconomic data [24]. Medical practitioners were benefitted by these findings, thereby reducing the dominance of opioid dependence.

3.5.7 Population-Level Mental Health Monitoring During Crises

During the COVID-19 pandemic, researchers evaluated the mental health patterns; researchers utilized data from the social media platform messages or posts and searches done by the people in search engines. Many instances related to fear, panic, melancholy, and observed restlessness were used to identify depression and anxiety in the subjects. Information related to resource allocation was achieved by identifying the regional variations in the effects on mental disorder [15]. These key findings acted as policymakers to proficiently distribute support resources and create public mental health campaigns.

3.5.8 ASD Genomic Data Predict Disorder

Genomic data were used by Simons Foundation Autism Research Initiative to identify genetic markers associated with ASD. GWAS data were subjected to ML techniques, which found ASD risk genes. The predictive accuracy of the approach used to identify ASD in high-risk families was 78% [27]. Families have been able to obtain behavioral therapy considerably sooner because of early genetic screening, which has improved developmental outcomes.

3.5.9 Posttraumatic Stress Disorder Risk Prediction

A prediction model has been implemented by the US Department of Veterans Affairs to identify returning soldiers who may be at risk for posttraumatic stress disorder (PTSD) [28]. Predeployment evaluations, battle exposure, and postdeployment medical records were all used in the model. In 85% of cases, the algorithm accurately predicted the likelihood of PTSD, allowing doctors to concentrate on high-risk patients. The intensity and chronicity of PTSD in impacted veterans were reduced by early therapy.

3.6 Challenges and Ethical Considerations in Predictive Analytics for Psychiatry

Although predictive analytics might change the area of psychiatry, implementing it raises ethical questions and has various challenges. Fixing these issues will help the technology's reliability, equality, and alignment with patient-centered care values. Some of the most significant moral conundrums and challenges brought forth by predictive analytics in mental health are presented below, along with the ethical issues and difficulties in predictive analytics.

3.6.1 Challenges or Difficulties in Predictive Analytics

Data Quality and Heterogeneity

Psychiatric datasets can include missing, incomplete, or noisy data due to the subjective character of mental health problems, dependence on self-reports, and variation in professional assessments; this presents a difficulty for prediction models. Unreliable forecasts thus show themselves as the means to lower model accuracy. For example, discrepancies might result from clinicians' different EHR symptom recording approaches [25].

Data Integration and Multimodal Complexity

Practical analysis depends on integrating psychiatric data from several sources. The sources of data that are discussed in the section above are wearable sensors, neuroimaging, and many others. Integrating the data is one of the technically challenging tasks, and it requires highly intricate and computational resources and robust frameworks. Probability of estimation of schizophrenia disease, for example, requires a combination of behavioral and neuroimaging data, which in turn requires high-level data reconciliation [13].

Algorithmic Biases

Unfair predictions by using ML approaches may be observed for groupings based on the sociographics of the healthcare recipients, i.e., the patients. Groupings based on income or groupings based on minorities (in terms of population sample) and majorities (in terms of population sample) may lead to groups being exemplified in disproportionate form. Such groupings can lead to model to misclassify the patient under consideration. For example, researchers have claimed that ML algorithm for depression prediction, which was trained on Western data, could not be generalized to the groups of non-Western populations [29].

Lack of Interpretability

Techniques or approaches based on DL operate as "black boxes." This makes it difficult to analyze how these techniques speculate mental health diseases. The predictive analytics might seem to be suboptimal if physicians lack the ability to act on outcome of the DL techniques being examined for disease prognosis. In one of the examples, a DL model predicts the risk of deliberate self-harming to end one's own life without an in-depth inspection of the speculation, which leads to lacking details [22].

Scalability and Resource Constraints

Low-resource organizations could struggle to deploy predictive analytics technologies due to a lack of accessible computing resources, trained staff, and necessary infrastructure. As a consequence, the disparity in access to mental healthcare between areas with rich and low incomes may worsen. For instance, researchers [23] said clinics with low resources would find it challenging to incorporate sophisticated AI-driven solutions.

Validation and Generalizability

The properties of real-world clinical data differ significantly from those of controlled research data; hence, predictive models built for the former may underperform those built for the latter. When models are applied to various groups, they may not work or even cause harm due to generalizability concerns. For instance, community-based care settings may be overlooked by a model trained on hospital data [24].

3.6.2 Ethical Considerations

Privacy and Confidentiality

Clinical notes and digital phenotyping data, which pertain to mental health, are extremely sensitive and necessitate stringent privacy safeguards, which impose an ethical conundrum/dilemma due to misuse of information, discrimination, or stigmatization that might result from data breaches. A patient's healthcare record could be at peril if noncompliant personnel gain access to their cognitive or mental health application information [29]. Following rules and regulations laid down by the Health Insurance Portability and Accountability Act and the General Data Protection Regulation will be facilitated to resolve this deontological conundrum. Leveraging secure data storage approaches and also using encryption to the patients data that are being stored can help diminish the privacy concerns.

Informed Consent

Patients, especially when using cutting-edge AI techniques, might not be entirely open about the intended use of patient information or data for predictive assessments, which develops yet another ethical complication, which may facilitate misinterpretation of information, which in turn may encourage either exploitation of information or a loss of trust. For example, patients using applications related to mental health may not be mindful that the third-party conglomerates are harnessing their health information for training the ML or DL algorithms [13]. One of the approaches for tackling this issue would be to inspire sincere and lucid communication about the gathering and utilization of information. Leveraging patient information with explicit and *a priori* approval of the patient can help dispose of the ethical obligation under consideration.

Risk of Overdiagnosis and Misdiagnosis

Another righteous obligation is that individuals under medical care may experience that they may be overdiagnosed or superfluously treated, which may be the result of excessive faith on AI-based approaches for prediction of health conditions. Hecen, an individual who is under medical care, could be agitated about the possibility of discrediting false positives or redundant medical treatment resulting from the predictions. For example, insufficient patient data may lead to a misclassification of a healthy patient being classified as unhealthy, as having a high risk of bipolar disease, by the ML or DL algorithm [22]. Hence, instead of trusting exclusively on ML or DL algorithm prognosis, the team of healthcare officials should try to use these ML and DL approaches or algorithms as a counterpart to solve the aforementioned ethical issue.

Equity and Accessibility

Yet, another ethical issue is the lack or scarcity of the resources in certain locations, which may hinder the equitable utilization to approaches pertaining to the healthcare predictive analytics. The potential elimination of unprivileged groups from leveraging the predictive analytics approaches may worsen the mental health treatment inequalities. Accessing the early diagnosis tools or devices might be challenging in places where the intricate healthcare frameworks are not available [24]. Handling such issues necessitates the requirement for building rationally priced remedies for underprivileged areas. Ensuring that the storage devices are capable of storing a large amount of people data to avoid excluding anyone can mitigate this ethical concern.

Accountability and Liability

The prediction systems, at times, may present false alarms (false positives); under such cases, one might be forced to imagine as to who should be held responsible for the false alarm that has been raised, ultimately whether it should be the coding personnel who should be held responsible or the medical practitioners or the organization of the healthcare. This remarks us with another moral and ethical issue. In such situations, the moral and lawful procedures become more complicated in relation to who is to be held accountable or responsible? Considering an example of a suicide prevention model that fails to find person at peril [23], the consequences that follow up would be unimaginable. Establishing open procedures for holding individuals responsible might help solve this problem and ensure models pass extensive testing and validation before anyone can use them.

Dehumanizing of Care

By putting statistics above humans, the moral dilemma of stressing too much about algorithms in mental healthcare has the potential to dehumanize patients. This causes questions about trust between the therapist and the patient, so that the therapeutic relationship may be in danger. To show the point, people might feel useless if doctors base treatment decisions exclusively on predictive analytics [29]. One might have to stress the requirement of physicians' involvement in comprehending and using forecasts to solve this issue.

3.7 Future Directions in Predictive Analytics for Psychiatry

Predictive analytics in psychiatry is quickly developing, thanks to advances in computer technology, ML, and data science. These discoveries are changing the diagnosis, treatment, and management of mental health problems. Nevertheless, additional advancements are required to fully address existing restrictions to utilize predictive analytics in mental health treatment. The most critical paths forward in this field are outlined here.

3.7.1 Precision Psychiatry

Precision psychiatry is based on customizing treatments to each person's specific combination of genetics, upbringing, and personality traits. The required advancements will be in merging genetic, neuroimaging, and behavioral information with other kinds of data to generate more exact and customized predictions. It is also vital to create adaptable models to monitor a patient's development and change. This would be reflected in improved treatment outcomes from tailored care paths made feasible by precision psychiatry. For example, few researchers [23] projected which MDD patients would react better to CBT than medication using neuroimaging and genetic data.

3.7.2 Real-Time Monitoring and Interventions

Digital technologies enabling real-time patient monitoring will become even more vital in the future of mental health treatment. Wearable technology and smartphone applications that track vital signs and other behavioral markers in real time will be the advances required. Improvements will also be needed with the analytics that alert doctors of significant real-time indicators of suicidal thoughts or a relapse. The result would be demonstrated to be a reduction in the possibility of abrupt catastrophes made possible by quick actions. For instance, using smartphones with sensors helps doctors quickly understand the speech patterns and social interactions of BPD patients [22].

3.7.3 AI-Powered Decision Support Systems

By arming clinicians with the tools they need to identify and treat mental health problems, AI in psychiatry will significantly improve clinical decision-making. Creating AI models that clinicians can comprehend and trust is an important step toward improving healthcare and utilizing currently established healthcare infrastructure, including EHR systems, to incorporate AI. This will make doctors' jobs easier and improve the precision of their diagnoses.

One example is AI-driven tools that may predict a patient's prognosis for treatment success using prior data and individual attributes [29].

3.7.4 Multimodal Data Integration

Combining data from several sources can help future models to be more accurate and whole. One area that needs improvement is the lack of a unified framework for integrating data from digital phenotyping, environmental factors, neuroimaging, and genetics. This also necessitates the development of new and better computational methods for dealing with diverse and massive datasets. This will significantly impact the complete understanding of mental health by illuminating the interplay of environmental, psychological, and biological elements. For instance, few researchers used fMRI, genetic data, and real-time behavioral tracking to predict the onset of schizophrenia [25].

3.7.5 Addressing Bias and Enhancing Generalizability

Future work must focus on making predictive analytics systems that are both inclusive and unbiased. There is a need to build datasets that reflect various racial and ethnic groupings, socioeconomic statuses, and geographical locations. Another requirement is implementing algorithms with built-in fairness measures to lessen the gap between demographic groups' projections. This is because it encourages fair access to predictive analytics benefits. One example is using mental health data from throughout the world to train algorithms; this way, they may be applied in both low- and high-income nations [24].

3.7.6 Ethical AI and Patient-Centric Models

Future work must put ethics first to keep patients' confidence and safety in predictive analytics for psychiatry. Advancements would be required with the following:

- The AI systems that are open and honest about how they arrived at their forecasts and how they follow ethical standards
- The methods for protecting the confidentiality of patient information and gathering their informed permission

The impact will be observed in protecting patients' rights and autonomy while fostering faith in prediction tools. For instance, AI models can help doctors and patients make informed decisions—by providing detailed explanations of predictions [29].

3.7.7 Decentralized and Secure Data Sharing

Boosting international research projects and increasing the scalability of predictive analytics depend on distributed and safe data-sharing technologies. Blockchain technology developments help make data exchange more transparent and safer. Using models trained on remote data using federated learning (FL) techniques helps avoid centralized storage of private data, which especially enables extensive research to be carried out in line with patient privacy protection. For example, researchers have presented that FL systems let mental health clinics worldwide cooperate without exchanging patient data [13].

3.7.8 Global Mental Health Applications

Predictive analytics will be very vital in aiding underprivileged areas with their mental health issues. Improvements are required for affordable scalable prediction systems that fit low-resource places and for teaching local doctors how to use these resources daily.

The effect of this improvement will be reducing inequalities in access to mental healthcare on a worldwide scale. For example, researchers cited the use of smartphone-based mental health screening tools in underserved rural areas where mental health practitioners are few [22].

3.7.9 Predictive Analytics in Prevention

Predictive analytics will be used to identify people at risk of developing mental health illnesses before symptoms appear as part of future efforts to prevent these disorders. The advancements are required for more research to fine-tune early-warning systems through longitudinal studies and using predictive modeling to find modifiable risk variables. This can effectively decrease healthcare expenditures in the long run by reorienting mental healthcare toward prevention rather than treatment. One example is the use of genetic and behavioral data to predict the risk of PTSD in individuals who work in high-stress industries, including the military [24].

3.7.10 Collaboration between Disciplines

Mental health practitioners, data scientists, ethicists, and legislators must work together for predictive analytics in psychiatry to have a bright future. There is need for the following:

- ➢ Programs that bring together experts from different fields help students learn technical and clinical skills.

3.7.11 Algorithm Creation and Deployment that Incorporates Multiple Perspectives

These advancements encourage new ideas while checking that existing predictive tools align with ethical and clinical requirements. For instance, research partnerships between healthcare institutions, tech corporations, and universities are an example of AI's potential use in psychiatry [23].

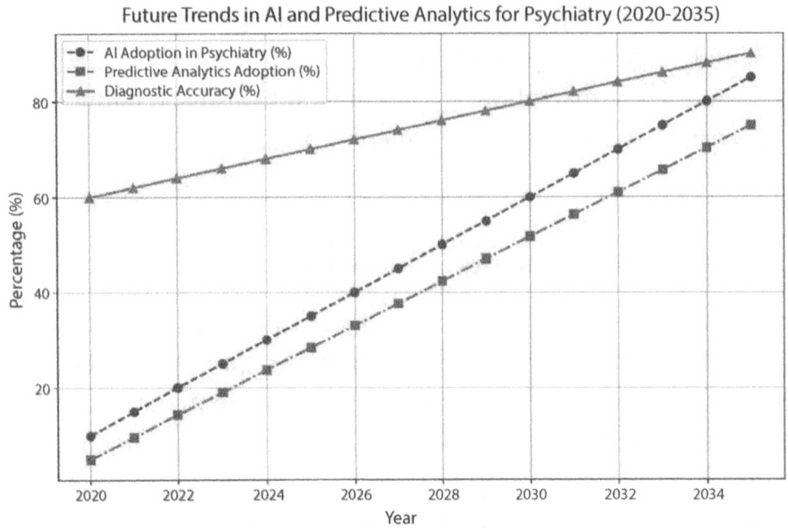

Figure 3.2 Future trends representation of AI and predictive analytics in psychiatry.

Trends that are predicted in AI adoption, implementation of predictive analytics, and improved accuracy in psychiatric diagnosis from 2020 to 2035 are given in Figure 3.2. Derived from the recent scholarly references, for instance, AI risk assessment tools are entering into psychiatric practice [30], digital therapeutics, and predictive models in treatment of schizophrenia and cognitive impairment detection [31]; AI and DL innovations are about to obliterate the paradigm of neuroimaging and psychiatric diagnostics [32].

This visual representation otherwise exhibits the predominant trend of increased AI co-opting and predictive analytics in mental health and seems to suggest that, in 2035, such technologies may yield tremendous improvement in diagnostic accuracy and treatment efficacy.

3.8 Conclusion

Big data analytics and predictive analytics in combination have facilitated a transformative era in the field of psychiatry. Deeper insights into the multifaceted aspect of mental health are explored by using wide-ranging sources of data, viz., EHRs, neuroimaging, digital phenotyping, and many others. The technologies driving big data analytics in psychiatry are changing at warp speed, thereby allowing researchers and clinicians to leverage these diverse datasets for better purposes. ML, NLP, neuroimaging tools, and cloud computing are the underlying drivers of such advancements, but digital phenotyping and visualization technologies provide actionable insights for real-time care. There are still other challenges such as data integration and ethical concerns that need to be addressed so that these technologies can be optimized to their potential. Predictive analytics is revolutionizing psychiatry in terms of making earlier diagnoses, personalizing treatment plans, and better patient outcomes. Applications in suicide prevention, relapse prediction, and treatment response bring it closer to revolutionizing mental healthcare. However, its challenges in the form of data quality, bias, and ethical concerns have to be overcome to reap all the benefits it promises. Predictive analytics is an interdisciplinary effort that will only keep improving with further advancements. The integration of predictive analytics in psychiatry has shown impressive real-world success across diverse applications, from early diagnosis to personalized treatment and public health monitoring. These case studies will show how the use of big data and advanced technologies can help improve mental health outcomes, save lives, and reduce healthcare costs. However, challenges such as algorithmic bias, data integration, and ethical concerns must be addressed to ensure equitable and effective implementation. Although predictive analytics has transforming potential in psychiatry, it is essential to address the challenges and ethical issues surrounding it to guarantee the suitable use of it. Predictive analytics emphasizes data quality, algorithm transparency, patient privacy, and the elimination of biases and accessibility issues, therefore helping to improve mental health results. To strike a balance between innovation and respect for patients' rights and dignity, it will be crucial to incorporate ethical concepts into the design and application of technology. With the advent of predictive analytics, psychiatry stands to gain access to mental healthcare that is proactive, individualized, and focused on the needs of the patient. Improving diagnostic precision and treatment efficacy are future goals of precision psychiatry, real-time monitoring, and integrated multimodal data. To reach these objectives, it must first overcome ethical obstacles, guarantee equal access, and encourage collaboration across disciplines. The field of mental health treatment could be revolutionized by predictive analytics with consistent innovation and careful application. A promising future lies ahead in the predictive analytics in psychiatry. Further transformations in mental healthcare can be seen by considering the developments that happen with real-time interventions, decentralized sharing of information, and ethical AI hold. By taking advantage of multidisciplinary collaboration and providing priorities to ethical details, the psychiatric domain can lead toward more proactive and healthcare recipient–centric approach that can enhance the psychological outcomes on a global scale.

Ultimately, although predictive analytics cannot replace human empathy and clinical judgment, it serves as a powerful tool to complement the expertise of mental health professionals, paving the way for a more efficient, personalized, and accessible psychiatric care system.

AI disclosure statement: The author acknowledges the use of AI-based tools for minor language editing or grammatical correction. However, all intellectual contributions, analyses, and conclusions presented in this chapter are entirely the author's own.

References

1. Insel, T.R. and Cuthbert, B.N., Medicine. Brain disorders? Precisely. *Science*, 348, 6234, 499–500, 2015.
2. Torous, J. and Roberts, L.W., The ethical use of mobile health technology in clinical psychiatry. *J. Nerv. Ment. Dis.*, 205, 1, 4–8, 2017.

3. Dhamala, E., Yeo, B.T.T., Holmes, A.J., One size does not fit all: Methodological considerations for brain-based predictive modeling in psychiatry. *Biol. Psychiatry*, 93, 8, 717–728, 2023.
4. Budisteanu, M., Papuc, S.M., Erbescu, A., Glangher, A., Andrei, E., Rad, F., Hinescu, M.E., Arghir, A., Review of structural neuroimaging and genetic findings in autism spectrum disorder–a clinical perspective. *Rev. Neurosci.*, 2024.
5. Torous, J., Kiang, M.V., Lorme, J., Onnela, J.-P., and others, New tools for new research in psychiatry: a scalable and customizable platform to empower data driven smartphone research. *JMIR Ment. Health*, 3, 2, e5165, 2016.
6. Sivarajkumar, S., Mohammad, H.A., Oniani, D., Roberts, K., Hersh, W., Liu, H., He, D., Visweswaran, S., Wang, Y., Clinical information retrieval: A literature review. *J. Healthcare Inf. Res.*, 1–40, 2024.
7. Georgiev, K., Wang, Y., Conkie, A., Sinclair, A., Christodoulou, V., Seyedzadeh, S., Price, M., Wales, A., Mills, N.L., Shenkin, S.D., McPeake, J., Fleuriot, J.D., Anand, A., Predicting incident dementia in community-dwelling older adults using primary and secondary care data from electronic health records. *Brain Commun.*, 7, 1, fcae469, 2024.
8. Li, Y.-T., Zhang, C., Han, J.-C., Shang, Y.-X., Chen, Z.-H., Cui, G.-B., Wang, W., Neuroimaging features of cognitive impairments in schizophrenia and major depressive disorder. *Ther. Adv. Psychopharmacol.*, 14, 20451253241243290, 2024.
9. Ripke, S., Neale, B.M., Corvin, A., Walters, J.T.R., Farh, K.-H., Holmans, P.A., Lee, P., Bulik-Sullivan, B., Collier, D.A., Huang, H., Pers, T.H., Agartz, I., Agerbo, E., Albus, M., Alexander, M., Amin, F., Bacanu, S.A., Begemann, M., Belliveau Jr., R.A., Bene, J., Bergen, S.E., Bevilacqua, E., Bigdeli, T.B., Black, D.W., Bruggeman, R., Buccola, N.G., Buckner, R.L., Byerley, W., Cahn, W., Cai, G., Campion, D., Cantor, R.M., Carr, V.J., Carrera, N., Catts, S.V., Chambert, K.D., Chan, R.C.K., Chen, R.Y.L., Chen, E.Y.H., Cheng, W., Cheung, E.F.C., Ann Chong, S., Robert Cloninger, C., Cohen, D., Cohen, N., Cormican, P., Craddock, N., Crowley, J.J., Curtis, D., Davidson, M., Davis, K.L., Degenhardt, F., Del Favero, J., Demontis, D., Dikeos, D., Dinan, T., Djurovic, S., Donohoe, G., Drapeau, E., Duan, J., Dudbridge, F., Durmishi, N., Eichhammer, P., Eriksson, J., Escott-Price, V., Essioux, L., Fanous, A.H., Farrell, M.S., Frank, J., Franke, L., Freedman, R.,

Freimer, N.B., Friedl, M., Friedman, J.I., Fromer, M., Genovese, G., Georgieva, L., Giegling, I., Giusti-Rodríguez, P., Godard, S., Goldstein, J.I., Golimbet, V., Gopal, S., Gratten, J., de Haan, L., Hammer, C., Hamshere, M.L., Hansen, M., Hansen, T., Haroutunian, V., Hartmann, A.M., Henskens, F.A., Herms, S., Hirschhorn, J.N., Hoffmann, P., Hofman, A., Hollegaard, M.V., Hougaard, D.M., Ikeda, M., Joa, I., Julià, A., Kahn, R.S., Kalaydjieva, L., Karachanak-Yankova, S., Karjalainen, J., Kavanagh, D., Keller, M.C., Kennedy, J.L., Khrunin, A., Kim, Y., Klovins, J., Knowles, J.A., Konte, B., Kucinskas, V., Ausrele Kucinskiene, Z., Kuzelova-Ptackova, H., Kähler, A.K., Laurent, C., Lee Chee Keong, J., Hong Lee, S., Legge, S.E., Lerer, B., Li, M., Li, T., Liang, K.-Y., Lieberman, J., Limborska, S., Loughland, C.M., Lubinski, J., Lönnqvist, J., Macek Jr., M., Magnusson, P.K.E., Maher, B.S., Maier, W., Mallet, J., Marsal, S., Mattheisen, M., Mattingsdal, M., McCarley, R.W., McDonald, C., McIntosh, A.M., Meier, S., Meijer, C.J., Melegh, B., Melle, I., Mesholam-Gately, R.I., Metspalu, A., Michie, P.T., Milani, L., Milanova, V., Mokrab, Y., Morris, D.W., Mors, O., Murphy, K.C., Murray, R.M., Myin-Germeys, I., Müller-Myhsok, B., Nelis, M., Nenadic, I., Nertney, D.A., Nestadt, G., Nicodemus, K.K., Nikitina-Zake, L., Nisenbaum, L., Nordin, A., O'Callaghan, E., O'Dushlaine, C., O'Neill, F.A., Oh, S.-Y., Olincy, A., Olsen, L., Van Os, J., Pantelis, C., Papadimitriou, G.N., Papiol, S., Parkhomenko, E., Pato, M.T., Paunio, T., Pejovic-Milovancevic, M., Perkins, D.O., Pietiläinen, O., Pimm, J., Pocklington, A.J., Powell, J., Price, A., Pulver, A.E., Purcell, S.M., Quested, D., Rasmussen, H.B., Reichenberg, A., Reimers, M.A., Richards, A.L., Roffman, J.L., Roussos, P., Ruderfer, D.M., Salomaa, V., Sanders, A.R., Schall, U., Schubert, C.R., Schulze, T.G., Schwab, S.G., Scolnick, E.M., Scott, R.J., Seidman, L.J., Shi, J., Sigurdsson, E., Silagadze, T., Silverman, J.M., Sim, K., Slominsky, P., Smoller, J.W., So, H.-C., Spencer, C.C.A., Stahl, E.A., Stefansson, H., Steinberg, S., Stogmann, E., Straub, R.E., Strengman, E., Strohmaier, J., Scott Stroup, T., Subramaniam, M., Suvisaari, J., Svrakic, D.M., Szatkiewicz, J.P., Söderman, E., Thirumalai, S., Toncheva, D., Tosato, S., Veijola, J., Waddington, J., Walsh, D., Wang, D., Wang, Q., Webb, B.T., Weiser, M., Wildenauer, D.B., Williams, N.M., Williams, S., Witt, S.H., Wolen, A.R., Wong, E.H.M., Wormley, B.K., Simon Xi, H., Zai, C.C., Zheng, X., Zimprich, F., Wray, N.R., Stefansson, K., Visscher,

P.M., Trust Case-Control Consortium, W., Adolfsson, R., Andreassen, O.A., Blackwood, D.H.R., Bramon, E., Buxbaum, J.D., Børglum, A.D., Cichon, S., Darvasi, A., Domenici, E., Ehrenreich, H., Esko, T., Gejman, P.V., Gill, M., Gurling, H., Hultman, C.M., Iwata, N., Jablensky, A.V., Jönsson, E.G., Kendler, K.S., Kirov, G., Knight, J., Lencz, T., Levinson, D.F., Li, Q.S., Liu, J., Malhotra, A.K., McCarroll, S.A., McQuillin, A., Moran, J.L., Mortensen, P.B., Mowry, B.J., Nöthen, M.M., Ophoff, R.A., Owen, M.J., Palotie, A., Pato, C.N., Petryshen, T.L., Posthuma, D., Rietschel, M., Riley, B.P., Rujescu, D., Sham, P.C., Sklar, P., St Clair, D., Weinberger, D.R., Wendland, J.R., Werge, T., Biological insights from 108 schizophrenia-associated genetic loci. *Nature*, 511, 7510, 421–427, 2014.

10. Thota, D., and others, Evaluating the relationship between fitbit sleep data and self-reported mood, sleep, and environmental contextual factors in healthy adults: Pilot observational cohort study. *JMIR Form. Res.*, 4, 9, e18086, 2020.
11. Cohrdes, C., Yenikent, S., Wu, J., Ghanem, B., Franco-Salvador, M., Vogelgesang, F., and others, Indications of depressive symptoms during the COVID-19 pandemic in Germany: Comparison of national survey and twitter data. *JMIR Ment. Health*, 8, 6, e27140, 2021.
12. Braithwaite, I., Zhang, S., Kirkbride, J.B., Osborn, D.P.J., Hayes, J.F., Air pollution (particulate matter) exposure and associations with depression, anxiety, bipolar, psychosis and suicide risk: A systematic review and meta-analysis. *Environ. Health Perspect.*, 127, 12, 126002, 2019.
13. Walsh, C.G., Ribeiro, J.D., Franklin, J.C., Predicting risk of suicide attempts over time through machine learning. *Clin. Psychol. Sci.*, 5, 3, 457–469, 2017.
14. Vieira, S., Pinaya, W.H.L., Mechelli, A., Using deep learning to investigate the neuroimaging correlates of psychiatric and neurological disorders: Methods and applications. *Neurosci. Biobehav. Rev.*, 74, 58–75, 2017.
15. De Choudhury, M., Pendse, S.R., Kumar, N., Benefits and harms of large language models in digital mental health, *arXiv preprint arXiv:2311.14693*, 2023.

16. Roza, T.H., Patusco, L.M., Zimerman, A., Ballester, P., Passos, I.C., Precision medicine in the assessment of suicide risk, in: *Precision Medicine for Investigators, Practitioners and Providers*, pp. 331–342, Elsevier, 2020. https://doi.org/10.1016/B978-0-12-819178-1.00032-0
17. Castro, V.M., Minnier, J., Murphy, S.N., Kohane, I., Churchill, S.E., Gainer, V., Cai, T., Hoffnagle, A.G., Dai, Y., Block, S., and others, Validation of electronic health record phenotyping of bipolar disorder cases and controls. *Am. J. Psychiatry*, 172, 4, 363–372, 2015.
18. Leaning, I.E., Ikani, N., Savage, H.S., Leow, A., Beckmann, C., Ruhé, H.G., Marquand, A.F., From smartphone data to clinically relevant predictions: A systematic review of digital phenotyping methods in depression. *Neurosci. Biobehav. Rev.*, 105541, 2024.
19. Webb, C.A., Trivedi, M.H., Cohen, Z.D., Dillon, D.G., Fournier, J.C., Goer, F., Fava, M., McGrath, P.J., Weissman, M., Parsey, R., and others, Personalized prediction of antidepressant v. placebo response: Evidence from the EMBARC study. *Psychol. Med.*, 49, 7, 1118–1127, 2019.
20. Mateos-Pérez, J.M., Dadar, M., Lacalle-Aurioles, M., Iturria-Medina, Y., Zeighami, Y., Evans, A.C., Structural neuroimaging as clinical predictor: A review of machine learning applications. *Neuroimage Clin.*, 20, 506–522, 2018.
21. Coppersmith, G., Leary, R., Crutchley, P., Fine, A., Natural language processing of social media as screening for suicide risk. *Biomed. Inf. Insights*, 10, 1178222618792860, 2018.
22. Faurholt-Jepsen, M., Frost, M., Ritz, C., Christensen, E.M., Jacoby, A.S., Mikkelsen, R.L., Knorr, U., Bardram, J.E., Vinberg, M., Kessing, L.V., Daily electronic self-monitoring in bipolar disorder using smartphones–the MONARCA I trial: a randomized, placebo-controlled, single-blind, parallel group trial. *Psychol. Med.*, 45, 13, 2691–2704, 2015.
23. Drysdale, A.T., Grosenick, L., Downar, J., Dunlop, K., Mansouri, F., Meng, Y., Fetcho, R.N., Zebley, B., Oathes, D.J., Etkin, A., and others, Resting-state connectivity biomarkers define neurophysiological subtypes of depression. *Nat. Med.*, 23, 1, 28–38, 2017.
24. Gomes, T., Tadrous, M., Mamdani, M.M., Paterson, J.M., Juurlink, D.N., The burden of opioid-related mortality in the United States. *JAMA Netw. Open*, 1, 2, e180217–e180217, 2018.

25. Penzel, N., Falkai, P., Koutsouleris, N., Kambeitz, J., F185. Brain structural patterns differentiate early-and late-onset cannabis use in psychotic patients: Preliminary results from the pronia study. *Schizophr. Bull.*, 44, Suppl 1, S293, 2018.
26. Zhang, Y., Wang, S., Hermann, A., Joly, R., Pathak, J., Development and validation of a machine learning algorithm for predicting the risk of postpartum depression among pregnant women. *J. Affect. Disord.*, 279, 1–8, 2021.
27. Sanders, S.J., He, X., Willsey, A.J., Ercan-Sencicek, A.G., Samocha, K.E., Cicek, A.E., Murtha, M.T., Bal, V.H., Bishop, S.L., Dong, S., and others, Insights into autism spectrum disorder genomic architecture and biology from 71 risk loci. *Neuron*, 87, 6, 1215–1233, 2015.
28. Ursano, R.J., Kessler, R.C., Stein, M.B., Naifeh, J.A., Aliaga, P.A., Fullerton, C.S., Wynn, G.H., Vegella, P.L., Ng, T.H.H., Zhang, B.G., and others, Risk factors, methods, and timing of suicide attempts among US Army soldiers. *JAMA Psychiatry*, 73, 7, 741–749, 2016.
29. Abbas, J., Wang, D., Su, Z., Ziapour, A., The role of social media in the advent of COVID-19 pandemic: crisis management, mental health challenges and implications. *Risk Manag. Healthc. Policy*, 1917–1932, 2021.
30. Islam, S., Shahriyar, R., Agarwala, A., Zaman, M., Ahamed, S., Rahman, R., Chowdhury, M.H., Sarker, F., Mamun, K.A., Artificial intelligence-based risk assessment tools for sexual, reproductive and mental health: a systematic review. *BMC Med. Inf. Decis. Making*, 25, 1, 132, 2025.
31. Sun, S., Li, C., Xie, X., Xianglong, W., Liu, T., Li, D., Duan, D., Yu, H., Wen, D., Digital Therapeutics for Cognitive Impairments Associated with Schizophrenia: Our Opinion. *Front. Psychiatry*, 16, 1535309, 2025.
32. Bansal, H., Jabalia, N., Shukla, K., Nautiyal, Y., Harnessing machine learning and deep learning techniques for neuroimaging, in: *Federated Learning for Neural Disorders in Healthcare 6.0*, Publisher is CRC Press, p. 158, 2025.

4

Effectiveness of Tele-Mental Health Services Provided by the Mental Health Professionals

Devyani Todi

Amity University, Kolkata, Allied and Behavioural Sciences, Saltlake, Kolkata, India

Abstract

Since the COVID-19 pandemic, there has been a significant increase in using tele-mental health services to increase accessibility among individuals who are unable to access it due to physical constraint. The aim of the current chapter is to examine the challenges faced by mental health professionals in providing services through tele-mental health services. We conducted a qualitative study to obtain key insights from the professionals. The initial pilot study involved interviewing 10 mental health professionals. The interview was conducted through Google Meet for approximately 1 hour for each session. A semistructured interview sheet was constructed in advance based on the current review of literature and gaps that have not been addressed. The present chapter is focused on exploring the key challenges that were faced by the mental health professionals while providing tele-mental health services and gaining insights on how these challenges can be addressed through digital platforms and interventions. Each interview was recorded and transcribed in verbatim and converted to a word document. Data analysis was conducted using thematic analysis and coding for each interview question. Finally, a model was constructed to explain the challenges and advantages of tele-mental health services. The findings indicate that 50% of mental health professionals believe that tele-mental health services are as effective as offline mode of providing the services. The results also highlight key challenges that are faced while using tele-mental health services, which are network issues, difficulty in rapport building and client engagement, difficulty understanding the body language, increased resistance from the client in expressing emotions, and poor client satisfaction with therapy.

***Keywords*:** Tele-mental health, qualitative study, mental health professionals

Email: devyanitodii58@gmail.com

Raghavendra M. Devadas, Vani Hiremani, Preethi, Praveen Gujjar, Sapna R. and Manoj Shettar (eds.) Psychiatry and Technology, (91–114) © 2026 Scrivener Publishing LLC

4.1 Introduction

Tele-mental health services have revolutionized the delivery of mental healthcare in India, offering an alternative to traditional in-person therapy. Online mental health services have emerged as a critical alternative to traditional in-person therapy, allowing mental health professionals to provide care remotely through various digital platforms. With the increasing burden of mental health disorders worldwide, exacerbated by the COVID-19 pandemic and barriers to in-person access, tele-mental health services have gained widespread acceptance. According to a systematic review by Varker *et al.* [1], tele-mental health interventions have demonstrated effectiveness comparable to in-person therapy, particularly for treating depression, anxiety, and posttraumatic stress disorder (PTSD).

The adoption of tele-mental health services has been driven by technological advancements, policy changes, and growing evidence supporting its efficacy. Research by the World Health Organization (WHO) [2] concluded that tele-mental health services not only improve patient engagement but also reduce hospitalization rates among individuals with chronic mental health conditions. A survey conducted by the American Psychological Association (APA) in 2021 found that 96% of psychologists who transitioned to telehealth during the pandemic intended to continue offering virtual services postpandemic, highlighting the long-term viability of remote mental healthcare. This chapter explores the scope, effectiveness, challenges, and future directions of tele-mental health services, focusing on their impact on patient well-being and mental health professionals' experiences.

The present chapter attempts to explore the effectiveness of tele-mental health services provided by mental health professionals. It examines their impact on patient outcomes, advantages and challenges, and future directions. The rising global demand for mental health services, coupled with advancements in digital technology, has made tele-mental health a critical area of research and practice.

Multiple findings have shown that remote mental health interventions can be as effective as face-to-face therapy for various conditions, including depression, anxiety, and PTSD. However, concerns regarding therapeutic relationships, digital access, and security persist.

This chapter aims to provide a comprehensive analysis of tele–mental health services, assessing their effectiveness and addressing the challenges mental health professionals face in this domain.

4.1.1 Definition and Scope

Tele–mental health refers to the use of telecommunications and digital technology to deliver mental health services remotely. These services encompass various forms, including video conferencing, phone calls, text-based counseling, and artificial intelligence (AI)–assisted therapy. WHO [3] has emphasized the role of tele–mental health in bridging the gap between demand and availability of mental healthcare, particularly in underserved populations.

With the growing demand for mental health services, especially in rural and remote areas, tele–mental health has expanded its scope to include various psychological interventions. These services are now being integrated into care settings, community well being programs, and even emergency psychiatric care, making it an essential component of modern mental health service delivery.

4.1.2 Modes of Delivery

Tele–mental health services are delivered through several modalities, each catering to different patient needs and technological access:

- **Video-based therapy**: Video conferencing enables real-time interactions, closely replicating traditional offline therapy. A study by Hull [4] found that patients receiving video-based cognitive behavioral therapy (CBT) showed significant symptom reduction in anxiety and depression, comparable to those undergoing face-to-face sessions.

- **Phone consultations**: This method is beneficial for individuals lacking internet access or requiring more flexible options. Research by Bashshur *et al.* [5] indicated that telephone-based therapy is effective for managing depression, with adherence rates comparable to in-person therapy.
- **Text-based therapy**: Conducted through messaging platforms and emails, this form of therapy allows asynchronous communication, particularly useful for individuals who prefer written expression. Studies have shown that text-based therapy can provide long-term psychological benefits, especially in cognitive behavioral interventions [6].
- **AI-powered support**: The emergence of AI-driven chatbots, such as Woebot, has provided preliminary psychological support to individuals experiencing mild to moderate symptoms of anxiety and depression. Andersson *et al.* [7] demonstrated that AI-assisted therapy can effectively reduce symptoms when used alongside traditional mental health interventions.

4.2 Effectiveness of Tele–Mental Health Services in Treating Specific Mental Health Disorders

Research has consistently demonstrated the efficacy of tele–mental health services in treating a wide range of mental health disorders. Tele–mental health interventions, delivered through video conferencing, phone calls, text-based counseling, and AI-assisted platforms, have been found to be effective. A meta-analysis by Spijkerman *et al.* [8] confirmed that tele–mental health interventions can significantly reduce symptoms of various mental health disorders, leading to improved patient outcomes and accessibility for individuals who might otherwise face barriers to treatment. Below is a detailed discussion of how tele–mental health has been applied effectively in the treatment of various psychiatric disorders: depression, anxiety disorders, PTSD, substance use disorders (SUDs), bipolar disorder, stress and burnout, and schizophrenia.

4.2.1 Depression

Depression is a prevalent mental health disorder, affecting globally 280 million people [3]. It is clinically defined by persistent feelings of low mood, lacking interest, fatigue, sleep disturbances, and cognitive impairments. Traditional face-to-face therapy has been the gold standard for managing depression, but tele–mental health has emerged as an effective alternative, especially for individuals with movement problems, financial constraints, or minimal access to in-person mental health services.

Multiple randomized controlled trials (RCTs) and meta-analyses have supported the effectiveness of tele–mental health for depression treatment. Andersson *et al.* [7] found that internet-based CBT produces outcomes similar to face-to-face CBT in reducing depressive symptoms. Another study by Bashshur *et al.* [9] showed that telephone-based therapy was effective in treating major depressive disorder, with patients demonstrating improvements in mood and functionality similar to those of patients receiving in-person therapy. Furthermore, Linardon *et al.* [10] examined the use of AI-driven chatbots, such as Woebot, in providing CBT for depression, concluding that these tools could significantly reduce symptoms in individuals experiencing mild to moderate depression.

The advantage of online mental health services for depression treatment is its ability to improve patient adherence. Studies indicate that patients are more likely to continue with therapy when they have remote access to care, reducing dropout rates compared to traditional therapy [11]. Tele–mental health also provides greater flexibility, allowing for more frequent follow-ups, crisis intervention, and real-time mood tracking, all of which contribute to improved clinical outcomes.

4.2.2 Anxiety Disorders

Anxiety disorders are among the most common psychiatric conditions treated *via* tele–mental health. Similar to depression, anxiety disorders respond well to remote interventions, particularly when therapy is structured and evidence-based.

A study [11] conducted a meta-analysis that included more than 30 studies comparing telehealth and in-person therapy for anxiety disorders. The findings indicated that tele–mental health was equally effective in reducing symptoms of anxiety, with video-based CBT and exposure therapy demonstrating the highest success rates. Internet-delivered exposure therapy has been particularly effective for conditions such as panic disorder and phobias [7].

A study by Shore *et al.* [12] highlighted the benefits of text-based therapy and asynchronous messaging for individuals with social anxiety disorder, as these methods allow patients to express themselves without the immediate pressure of face-to-face interaction. Patients with severe anxiety symptoms may find virtual therapy less intimidating than in-person sessions, making them more likely to seek and continue treatment.

Tele–mental health also plays a significant role in treating anxiety-related sleep disturbances. Wagner *et al.* [13] found that online mindfulness-based interventions significantly reduced symptoms of insomnia and anxiety, helping patients regulate their sleep cycles and reduce stress.

4.2.3 Substance Use Disorders

SUDs, including alcohol use disorder and opioid addiction, are complex conditions that require long-term behavioral therapy, medication management, and relapse prevention strategies. Tele–mental health has emerged as a critical tool in addiction treatment, particularly for individuals in rural areas or those unable to attend in-person rehabilitation programs.

A study [14] found that tele–mental health significantly reduces relapse rates by increasing access to support groups, counseling, and medication-assisted treatment for opioid dependence. Telehealth programs using video therapy and mobile applications have shown success in tracking patient progress, monitoring medication adherence, and providing 24/7 crisis support.

A growing number of digital recovery programs, such as text-based support groups and AI-driven relapse prevention tools, have also been integrated into tele–mental health models. These programs offer real-time motivational interventions, helping patients maintain long-term sobriety.

4.2.4 Posttraumatic Stress Disorder

PTSD is a psychiatric problem that develops after experiencing traumatic events such as sexual assault, natural disasters, or life-threatening experiences. Symptoms include flashbacks, nightmares, hypervigilance, emotional numbness, and avoidance behaviors.

The Veterans Affairs (VA) Tele–Mental Health Program has played a pioneering role in using telehealth to treat PTSD. A study [15] evaluated the effectiveness of video-based prolonged exposure therapy for veterans with PTSD, finding that remote therapy was just as effective as in-person treatment in reducing PTSD symptoms.

Another study [16] reviewed RCTs comparing telehealth PTSD treatment with traditional therapy and found that virtual interventions were highly effective, particularly when structured therapies such as cognitive processing therapy and trauma-focused CBT were used.

One of the key advantages of tele–mental health in PTSD treatment is its ability to reach trauma survivors in remote areas and provide continuous follow-up care. Many PTSD patients struggle with agoraphobia or hypervigilance, making it difficult to attend in-person therapy. Tele–mental health provides a safe and controlled environment for them to engage in therapy.

4.2.5 Bipolar Disorder

Bipolar disorder is a persistent mood disorder that includes episodes of mania and depression. Tele-mental health has proven effective in managing mood instability, preventing relapses, and providing psychoeducation.

A study by Varker *et al.* [17] found that telepsychiatry was effective in stabilizing patients with bipolar disorder, particularly in cases where frequent monitoring and medication adjustments were required. Telehealth platforms allow psychiatrists to conduct real-time mood assessments and adjust treatment plans accordingly.

Patients with bipolar disorder often benefit from digital CBT, online mood tracking tools, and mobile reminders for medication adherence. These digital tools provide continuous mood monitoring, helping patients recognize early warning signs of mood episodes.

4.2.6 Stress and Burnout

Work-related stress and burnout have increased significantly in recent years, especially among healthcare professionals, corporate employees, and frontline workers. Tele-mental health has been widely used to provide stress management programs, resilience training, and online mindfulness interventions.

A study [16] found that online mindfulness therapy effectively reduced stress levels and improved overall well-being. Telehealth platforms offering virtual coaching and stress reduction techniques have also been successful in preventing burnout and improving work–life balance.

4.2.7 Schizophrenia and Other Severe Mental Illnesses

Schizophrenia and other psychotic disorders require ongoing psychiatric care, medication management, and psychosocial support. A study [17] found that tele-mental health improved access to psychiatric services for individuals with schizophrenia, particularly those in rural and underserved areas.

Telepsychiatry has been successful in reducing hospitalization rates, improving medication adherence, and providing family education. Patients with schizophrenia who receive telehealth interventions show fewer relapses and improved daily functioning compared to those relying solely on in-person care.

4.3 Conceptual and Theoretical Foundations of Tele–Mental Health

The effectiveness of tele–mental health interventions is rooted in various psychological and therapeutic frameworks that have been adapted to digital platforms. One of the most prominent models supporting tele–mental health is CBT, which has been successfully delivered *via* online sessions, mobile applications, and automated chatbots. A study [18] found that internet-based CBT yielded outcomes comparable to in-person therapy in the treatment of generalized anxiety disorder and depression, demonstrating its adaptability to virtual formats. Another widely used theoretical model is dialectical behavior therapy (DBT), which has been effectively implemented in telehealth settings to assist individuals with borderline personality disorder and emotional dysregulation. It was reported that [19] remote DBT interventions contributed to significant reductions in self-harm behaviors and suicidal ideation among patients, highlighting the feasibility of tele-based skills training and crisis interventions.

Person-centered therapy, which emphasizes the importance of empathy, congruence, and unconditional positive regard, has also been adapted to tele–mental health platforms. While some researchers argue that virtual therapy may weaken the therapeutic alliance due to limited nonverbal communication, Simpson *et al.* [14] found that 85% of patients in teletherapy reported feeling connected to their therapist, suggesting that a strong therapeutic bond can still be cultivated through digital means. Furthermore, the rise of mindfulness-based interventions in tele–mental health, facilitated through mobile applications and virtual coaching, has led to promising results in stress reduction, emotional regulation, and cognitive flexibility [13]. The integration of these evidence-based therapeutic approaches into tele–mental health services supports its efficacy and underscores the potential for continued innovation in digital mental healthcare.

4.4 Effectiveness of Tele–Mental Health Services: Empirical Evidence

Tele–mental health services have been rigorously examined through meta-analyses, RCTs, and real-world case studies to assess their comparative effectiveness, patient satisfaction, and success rates in treating various mental health conditions.

4.4.1 Comparative Effectiveness versus In-Person Therapy

Several meta-analyses have confirmed that tele–mental health interventions yield outcomes comparable to in-person therapy. A study [8] analyzed multiple studies on digital mental health interventions and found no significant differences in effectiveness between online therapy and offline sessions. This conclusion agrees with the findings from Turgoose *et al.* [11], who conducted RCTs for depression, anxiety, and PTSD treatment, demonstrating that telehealth interventions resulted in similar symptom reductions as in-person therapy. Furthermore, research indicates that the convenience and accessibility of remote therapy contribute to higher patient retention rates compared to conventional settings.

4.4.2 Patient Satisfaction and Engagement

Studies on user adherence and therapeutic alliance in remote therapy suggest that patients report high levels of satisfaction with tele–mental health services. Another study found that more than 80% of patients felt their therapeutic relationship remained strong despite virtual sessions. Additionally, the psychological comfort of accessing therapy from one's home has been cited as a key factor in engagement and continued participation in mental health programs. This is particularly significant for individuals experiencing social anxiety, agoraphobia, or mobility constraint.

4.4.3 Success Rates in Treating Specific Mental Health Disorders

Empirical evidence supports the effectiveness of tele–mental health in treating a variety of psychiatric conditions. It was Spijkerman *et al.* [8] who demonstrated that internet-based CBT successfully reduced symptoms of depression and anxiety. A study [15] found that veterans receiving virtual PTSD therapy reported improvements comparable to those attending in-person sessions. Similarly, Bashshur *et al.* [5] concluded that telehealth interventions were effective in treating SUDs, whereas Shore *et al.* [12] showed that digital platforms improved treatment accessibility for individuals.

4.5 Effectiveness of Tele–Mental Health Services According to Mental Health Professionals

4.5.1 Difficulties in Building Therapeutic Rapport and Observing Nonverbal Cues

One of the most common concerns expressed by therapists is the difficulty of establishing and maintaining a strong therapeutic alliance in remote settings, particularly for first-time therapy clients. Research suggests that the therapeutic relationship is one of the most significant predictors of positive mental health outcomes, and some clinicians worry that video-based interactions may lack the warmth and presence of in-person communication.

Furthermore, nonverbal cues—such as body language, microexpressions, and subtle behavioral changes—are more challenging to perceive through a screen. Many therapists, particularly those practicing psychodynamic or body-focused therapies, report that these limitations can hinder their ability to make accurate assessments. A clinical psychologist specializing in trauma therapy shared that telehealth has made it harder to detect dissociative symptoms in her clients, as subtle changes in facial expressions or posture might go unnoticed.

4.5.2 Challenges in Crisis Management and Risk Assessment

Crisis intervention presents another significant challenge for tele-mental health providers. In face-to-face settings, a therapist can assess a client's immediate risk more effectively and take action if needed, such as contacting emergency services or physically intervening in cases of self-harm or suicidal ideation. However, in remote therapy, the therapist has limited control over the client's environment, making real-time crisis intervention more complex.

Mental health professionals working with high-risk populations, such as those experiencing suicidal ideation or severe psychosis, often express concerns about their ability to provide adequate support remotely. Many therapists report feeling uneasy about conducting suicide risk assessments virtually, as they cannot ensure immediate safety measures if a client is in distress. Some organizations have addressed this challenge by implementing structured emergency protocols, including identifying a client's location at the start of each session and having local emergency contacts on file. However, the lack of standardized crisis management strategies in teletherapy remains an area of concern among professionals.

4.5.3 Technological Barriers and Client Engagement Issues

Although tele-mental health increases accessibility for many, it also introduces new challenges related to technology. Therapists working with older adults, individuals from lower socioeconomic backgrounds, or those with cognitive impairments report that technological barriers—such as lack of access to a stable internet connection, unfamiliarity with digital platforms, or difficulty navigating online systems—can hinder effective treatment.

Moreover, some clients struggle with maintaining focus during remote sessions. Unlike in a therapy office, where distractions are minimized, home environments may have interruptions such as background noise, family members, or connectivity issues that disrupt the therapeutic process. Some clinicians have also noted that clients who struggle with engagement in traditional therapy settings may be more prone to avoidance behaviors in teletherapy, such as turning off their camera, multitasking, or disengaging from the conversation.

4.6 Challenges Faced by Mental Health Professionals While Using Tele–Mental Health Services

While tele–mental health services have expanded access to mental healthcare, mental health professionals encounter several challenges that impact the quality and efficacy of remote interventions. These challenges include difficulties in building therapeutic rapport, limitations in nonverbal communication, crisis management concerns, technological and accessibility barriers, ethical and confidentiality risks, and regulatory issues.

One of the primary concerns experienced by professionals is the difficulty in establishing and maintaining a strong therapeutic alliance in virtual settings. The therapeutic relationship is a crucial factor in successful treatment outcomes, yet the lack of physical presence and reliance on digital interfaces can make it harder for clinicians to build trust, particularly with new clients. Research [16] suggests that there is difficulty in reading nonverbal cues, which can lead to a perceived lack of warmth, making it difficult for some clients to fully engage in therapy. Therapists also note that certain psychodynamic and humanistic approaches, which rely heavily on nonverbal cues and the therapist's physical presence, may be less effective in telehealth formats.

Limitations in nonverbal communication pose another significant challenge. Many clinicians rely on subtle facial expressions, posture, and behavioral cues to assess their clients' emotional states, which may be less perceptible. A study [10] highlights that tele–mental health reduces the therapist's ability to observe microexpressions or sudden behavioral shifts, potentially affecting diagnostic accuracy, particularly for conditions such as autism spectrum disorder or schizophrenia. Additionally, some clients may feel uncomfortable being on camera, further limiting the therapist's ability to assess visual cues.

Crisis management and risk assessment are major concerns among mental health professionals, particularly when working with clients experiencing severe distress, suicidal ideation, or psychosis. In face-to-face settings, a therapist can assess immediate risk more effectively and intervene directly if necessary. However, in a virtual setting, ensuring the safety of a client becomes more complex. It was [17] found that therapists reported heightened anxiety about conducting suicide risk assessments *via* telehealth, as they cannot physically intervene in emergencies. Although some professionals implement safety protocols, such as requiring clients to share their physical location at the start of a session or having emergency contacts readily available, the lack of direct control over the client's environment remains a critical challenge.

Technological and accessibility barriers further complicate the effectiveness of tele–mental health services. Not all clients have access to a stable internet connection, a private space for therapy, or the technical proficiency to navigate telehealth platforms. A study [5] found that older adults, individuals from lower-income backgrounds, and those with cognitive impairments often face difficulties in accessing virtual therapy, leading to higher dropout rates. Moreover, therapists also face technical issues such as connectivity disruptions, software malfunctions, and security concerns that can interrupt sessions and impact the flow of therapy.

Ethical and confidentiality risks are another critical challenge for mental health professionals using telehealth platforms. Ensuring client privacy in remote settings can be difficult, particularly for individuals in abusive households or those without a private space to conduct therapy sessions. A study by Hilty *et al.* [18] found that therapists working with survivors of domestic abuse reported concerns about clients being overheard by abusers during virtual sessions, limiting their ability to speak freely. Additionally, the reliance on digital platforms raises concerns about data security, as telehealth services are vulnerable to breaches despite encryption efforts.

Finally, legal and regulatory challenges further complicate the implementation of tele–mental health. Licensing restrictions often require therapists to have a license, limiting their ability to provide care across borders. In a study [16], it was noted that inconsistent regulations across jurisdictions create administrative burdens for clinicians, restricting the scalability of tele–mental health services. Additionally, concerns regarding insurance reimbursement, liability in teletherapy, and the need for standardized best practices further add to the difficulties faced by professionals in this domain.

Despite these challenges, mental health professionals continue to adapt to tele–mental health by integrating innovative strategies such as hybrid therapy models, digital literacy training for clients, and the use of AI-driven tools for remote assessment. Although tele–mental health remains an essential tool in modern psychological care, addressing these limitations through policy reforms, technological advancements, and clinician training will be critical in ensuring its long-term effectiveness.

4.7 Tele–Mental Health for Children and Adolescents

Research suggests that tele–mental health can be effective for treating various psychological conditions in children and adolescents, including anxiety, depression, attention-deficit/hyperactivity disorder, and PTSD. A meta-analysis by Myers *et al.* [19] found that telehealth-based CBT for children with anxiety disorders was equally effective as in-person therapy. Similarly, a study by Comer *et al.* [20] indicated that teletherapy interventions for youth with PTSD led to significant symptom reduction and were well-received by both children and caregivers.

One of the main advantages of tele–mental health for young populations is its ability to reduce barriers to access. Many children and adolescents, particularly those living in rural areas or in communities with a shortage of mental health professionals, have benefited from teletherapy services that allow them to receive treatment from the comfort of their homes. Furthermore, telehealth might help in reducing resistance and stigma, as young individuals can engage in therapy privately without concerns about being judged by peers.

Moreover, school-based tele–mental health programs have been particularly effective in reaching children who might otherwise lack access to care. A review [21] found that integrating tele–mental health services into schools improved behavioral and academic outcomes, as well as overall mental well-being. These programs facilitate early intervention, allowing school counselors and therapists to identify and address issues such as bullying, social anxiety, and learning disabilities before they escalate.

Challenges faced in tele–mental health for children and adolescents

Despite its effectiveness, mental health professionals face several challenges when implementing tele–mental health services for children and adolescents.

4.7.1 Engagement and Attention Span

Children, particularly younger ones, may have difficulty maintaining focus during virtual therapy sessions. Unlike adults, children often require interactive and play-based therapeutic techniques, which may be harder to implement in a virtual format. Studies have shown that younger children are more likely to disengage or become distracted during teletherapy sessions, leading to reduced treatment efficacy [21]. To address this, therapists often incorporate interactive elements such as digital games, drawing activities, or storytelling to maintain engagement.

4.7.2 Developmental Considerations

Therapeutic approaches must be tailored to the child's developmental stage. Adolescents may benefit more from traditional talk therapy *via* telehealth, whereas younger children may require more visual and interactive strategies. Additionally, younger children may struggle with understanding abstract concepts conveyed through a screen, requiring therapists to adapt their communication styles accordingly. Research by Boydell *et al.* [23] highlights that clinicians working with young children through telehealth must modify their usual interventions to fit the limitations of digital interactions.

4.7.3 Parental Involvement and Privacy Concerns

The role of parents in tele–mental health services for children and adolescents is crucial. Younger children often require parental involvement to facilitate therapy sessions, help with technology, and reinforce therapeutic strategies at home. However, parental engagement can also introduce challenges, particularly if there are conflicts within the family, lack of parental support, or concerns about privacy. Adolescents, in particular, may be reluctant to engage in therapy if they feel their confidentiality is at risk. Studies have found that some teens prefer in-person sessions to ensure their discussions remain private from family members [24]. To address this, therapists must establish clear confidentiality agreements and help adolescents create private spaces for virtual sessions.

4.7.4 Crisis Management and Risk Assessment

Managing mental health crises remotely is particularly challenging with children and adolescents. If a young client exhibits suicidal ideation or self-harming behavior, the therapist has limited ability to intervene directly. A study [25] found that therapists providing tele–mental health services to at-risk youth reported increased stress due to concerns about their inability to ensure the child's immediate safety. To mitigate risks, many practitioners implement safety protocols, such as identifying emergency contacts at the beginning of treatment, working closely with caregivers, and developing crisis response plans tailored to the child's needs.

4.7.5 Technological Barriers and Digital Inequality

Access to reliable technology is another significant challenge in tele-mental health for children and adolescents. Whereas many families have internet access, others—particularly those from low-income backgrounds—may struggle with unstable connections, lack of access to a private space, or unfamiliarity with telehealth platforms. Research [26] indicates that disparities in access to digital resources can create inequities in mental healthcare, with some children receiving lower-quality or inconsistent treatment due to technological limitations. Addressing this issue requires systemic efforts to improve digital accessibility and provide alternative support options for those without reliable technology.

4.8 Ethical and Legal Considerations

Mental health professionals must also navigate ethical and legal complexities in tele-mental health for children and adolescents. Licensing laws often restrict therapists from providing care across state or national borders, limiting the availability of specialists for certain populations [27]. Additionally, data security is a concern, as ensuring compliance with privacy laws such as the Health Insurance Portability and Accountability Act and the Children's Online Privacy Protection Act is essential when working with minors.

4.9 Case Studies and Real-World Applications

Real-world applications highlight the success of tele-mental health in various settings. The VA Tele-Mental Health Program has demonstrated improved PTSD management among veterans. University-based teletherapy programs have effectively addressed student mental health needs. Corporate telehealth solutions have enhanced workplace mental well-being, reducing stress and burnout among employees.

4.10 Future Directions and Innovations

Advancements in AI, wearable technology, and policy frameworks will continue to shape the future of tele–mental health. AI-driven mental health chatbots, such as Woebot and Wysa, are expected to play an increasingly significant role in providing preliminary psychological support [28]. The integration of wearable devices for real-time mood tracking and biofeedback interventions has also been explored demonstrating the effectiveness of smart technology in enhancing mental health self-monitoring. Additionally, policy standardization by organizations such as the APA and WHO will be essential in ensuring the ethical and equitable expansion of tele–mental health services.

Despite these challenges, mental health professionals widely agree that tele–mental health is here to stay and will continue to play a crucial role in modern psychological care. Many advocate for a hybrid model—combining in-person and remote therapy—to maximize accessibility while addressing the limitations of virtual sessions. This approach allows clients to receive teletherapy when convenient but also attend face-to-face sessions when deeper assessment, crisis intervention, or enhanced therapeutic connection is needed.

Additionally, continued training for mental health professionals on best practices for remote therapy is essential. Many therapists have adapted their communication strategies to enhance engagement in virtual sessions, such as using more verbal affirmations, checking in more frequently on a client's emotional state, and adjusting their therapeutic approaches to fit the digital medium.

Technological advancements, such as AI-assisted mental health tools and virtual reality therapy, may further enhance the effectiveness of remote interventions. Some clinicians have expressed optimism about AI-driven assessment tools that can analyze speech patterns and microexpressions to provide additional diagnostic insights in virtual settings.

AI disclosure statement: The author acknowledges the use of AI-based tools for minor language editing or grammatical correction. However, all intellectual contributions, analyses, and conclusions presented in this chapter are entirely the author's own.

Bibliography

1. Varker, T., Brand, R.M., Ward, J., Terhaag, S., Phelps, A., Efficacy of telepsychology interventions for people with anxiety, depression, post-traumatic stress disorder, and adjustment disorder: A systematic review and meta-analysis. *Psychol. Serv.*, *16*, 4, 585–599, 2019, https://doi.org/10.1037/ser0000234.
2. World Health Organization (WHO), Guidelines on digital health interventions for health system strengthening, WHO, 2020, https://www.who.int/publications/i/item/9789241550505.
3. Mohr, D.C., Ho, J., Duffecy, J., Baron, K.G., Lehman, K.A., Jin, L., Reifler, D., Perceived barriers to psychological treatments and their relationship to depression. *J. Clin. Psychol.*, *68*, 4, 437–450, 2012, https://doi.org/10.1002/jclp.20862.
4. Hull, T.D., Text-based mental health interventions: A review of the literature and implications for practice. *J. Technol. Hum. Serv.*, *33*, 3, 267–281, 2015, https://doi.org/10.1080/15228835.2015.1063170.
5. Bashshur, R.L., Shannon, G.W., Bashshur, N., Yellowlees, P.M., The empirical evidence for telemedicine interventions in mental disorders. *Telemed. e-Health*, *22*, 2, 87–113, 2016, https://doi.org/10.1089/tmj.2015.0206.
6. Luo, C., Sanger, N., Singhal, N., Pattrick, K., Shams, I., Shahid, H., Hoang, P., Schmidt, J., Lee, J., Haber, S., Puckering, M., Buchanan, N., Lee, P., Ng, K., Sun, S., Kheyson, S., Chung, D.C.Y., Sanger, S., Thabane, L., Samaan, Z., A comparison of electronically-delivered and face-to-face cognitive behavioural therapies in depressive disorders: A systematic review and meta-analysis. *EClinicalMedicine*, *24*, 100442, 2020, https://doi.org/10.1016/j.eclinm.2020.100442.
7. Andersson, G., Cuijpers, P., Carlbring, P., Riper, H., Hedman, E., Guided internet-based vs. face-to-face cognitive behavior therapy for psychiatric and somatic disorders: A systematic review and

meta-analysis. *World Psychiatry*, *13*, 3, 288–295, 2014, https://doi.org/10.1002/wps.20151.
8. Spijkerman, M.P.J., Pots, W.T.M., Bohlmeijer, E.T., Effectiveness of online mindfulness-based interventions in improving mental health: A review and meta-analysis. *Clin. Psychol. Rev.*, *45*, 102–114, 2016, https://doi.org/10.1016/j.cpr.2016.03.009.
9. Bashshur, R., Shannon, G., Krupinski, E., Grigsby, J., The empirical foundations of telemedicine interventions in primary care. *Telemed. e-Health*, *22*, 5, 342–375, 2016, https://doi.org/10.1089/tmj.2016.0045.
10. Linardon, J., Cuijpers, P., Carlbring, P., Messer, M., Fuller-Tyszkiewicz, M., The efficacy of internet-based cognitive-behavioral therapy for psychiatric disorders: A meta-analysis of randomized controlled trials. *Psychol. Bull.*, *145*, 9, 943–972, 2019, https://doi.org/10.1037/bul0000194.
11. Turgoose, D., Ashwick, R., Murphy, D., Systematic review of lessons learned from delivering teletherapy to veterans with post-traumatic stress disorder. *BMJ Open*, *8*, 4, e019265, 2018, https://doi.org/10.1136/bmjopen-2017-019265.
12. Shore, J.H., Yellowlees, P., Caudill, R., Johnston, B., Turvey, C., Mishkind, M., Krupinski, E., Myers, K., Shore, P., Kaftarian, E., Best practices in videoconferencing-based telemental health. *Telemed. e-Health*, *24*, 3, 163–169, 2018, https://doi.org/10.1089/tmj.2017.0177.
13. Wagner, B., Horn, A.B., Maercker, A., Internet-based versus face-to-face cognitive-behavioral intervention for depression: A randomized controlled trial. *J. Affective Disord.*, *126*, 1-2, 43–52, 2020, https://doi.org/10.1016/j.jad.2010.12.001.
14. Simpson, S.G. and Reid, C.L., Therapeutic alliance in videoconferencing psychotherapy: A systematic review. *Clin. Psychol. Psychother.*, *28*, 2, 276–289, 2021, https://doi.org/10.1002/cpp.2524.
15. Luxton, D.D., Pruitt, L.D., O'Brien, K., Kramer, G., An evaluation of the feasibility and safety of a home-based telemental health treatment for posttraumatic stress in veterans. *Psychol. Serv.*, *13*, 2, 119–127, 2016, https://doi.org/10.1037/ser0000061.
16. Wind, T.R., Rijkeboer, M., Andersson, G., Riper, H., The COVID-19 pandemic: The 'black swan' for mental health care and a turning point for e-health. *Internet Interventions*, *20*, 100317, 2020, https://doi.org/10.1016/j.invent.2020.100317.

17. Varker, T., Brand, R.M., Ward, J., Terhaag, S., Phelps, A., Efficacy of telehealth interventions for PTSD: A rapid evidence assessment. *BMC Psychiatry*, *19*, 1, 1–11, 2019, https://doi.org/10.1186/s12888-019-2150-6.
18. Hilty, D.M., Ferrer, D.C., Parish, M.B., Johnston, B., Callahan, E.J., Yellowlees, P.M., The effectiveness of tele-mental health: A 2013 review. *Telemed. e-Health*, *19*, 6, 444–454, 2013, https://doi.org/10.1089/tmj.2013.0075.
19. Myers, K., Nelson, E.-L., Rabinowitz, T., Hilty, D., Baker, D., Barnwell, S., American Telemedicine Association practice guidelines for telemental health with children and adolescents. *Telemed. e-Health*, *23*, 10, 779–804, 2017, https://doi.org/10.1089/tmj.2017.0177.
20. Comer, J.S., Furr, J.M., Kerns, C.E., Miguel, E., Coxe, S., Elkins, R.M., Kendall, P.C., Internet-delivered, family-based treatment for early-onset OCD: A pilot randomized trial. *J. Consult. Clin. Psychol.*, *83*, 5, 965–973, 2015, https://doi.org/10.1037/ccp0000028.
21. Spaulding, R., Belz, N., DeLurgio, S.A., Williams, D.K., Evaluation of a telepsychiatry pilot project: Patient satisfaction and provider acceptability. *J. Telemed. Telecare*, *16*, 2, 103–107, 2010, https://doi.org/10.1258/jtt.2009.090906.
22. Gloff, N.E., LeNoue, S.R., Novins, D.K., Myers, K., Telemental health for children and adolescents. *Int. Rev. Psychiatry*, *27*, 6, 513–524, 2015, https://doi.org/10.3109/09540261.2015.1086322.
23. Boydell, K.M., Hodgins, M., Pignatiello, A., Teshima, J., Edwards, H., Willis, D., Using technology to deliver mental health services to children and youth: A scoping review. *J. Can. Acad. Child Adolesc. Psychiatry*, *23*, 2, 87–99, 2014.
24. Nelson, E.-L., Cain, S., Sharp, S., Considerations for telehealth use with children and adolescents. *Child Adolesc. Psychiatr. Clin. North Am.*, *31*, 1, 27–40, 2022, https://doi.org/10.1016/j.chc.2021.08.008.
25. Keesara, S., Jonas, A., Schulman, K., Covid-19 and health care's digital revolution. *N. Engl. J. Med.*, *382*, 23, e82, 2020, https://doi.org/10.1056/NEJMp2005835.
26. Goldschmidt, K., The COVID-19 pandemic: Technology use to support the wellbeing of children. *J. Pediatr. Nurs.*, *53*, 88–90, 2020, https://doi.org/10.1016/j.pedn.2020.04.013.

27. Fitzpatrick, K.K., Darcy, A., Vierhile, M., Delivering cognitive behavior therapy to young adults with symptoms of depression and anxiety using a fully automated conversational agent (Woebot): A randomized controlled trial. *JMIR Mental Health*, *4*, 2, e19, 2017, https://doi.org/10.2196/mental.7785.
28. Koonin, L.M., Hoots, B., Tsang, C.A., Leroy, Z., Farris, K., Jolly, B., Harris, A.M., Trends in the use of telehealth during the emergence of the COVID-19 pandemic—United States, January–March 2020. *Morb. Mortal. Wkly. Rep.*, *69*, 43, 1595–1599, 2020, https://doi.org/10.15585/mmwr.mm6943a3.
29. Norwood, C., Moghaddam, N., Malins, S., Sabin-Farrell, R., Working alliance and outcome effectiveness in e-therapy for mental health: A systematic review and meta-analysis. *PLoS One*, *13*, 9, e0203085, 2018, https://doi.org/10.1371/journal.pone.0203085.

5

Therapeutic Alliance and Effectiveness of Digital Mental Health Interventions

Mihna A. Arakkal[1] and M. Rejoyson Thangal[2]*

[1]Department of Humanities and Social Sciences, Indian Institute of Technology, Dhanbad, India
[2]Department of Psychology, Pondicherry University, Puducherry, India

Abstract
Digital mental health interventions (DMHIs) are technology-driven approaches such as smartphone applications, web-based programs, virtual reality, wearable devices, and video games for the promotion, prevention, education, assessment, and treatment related to mental health problems. Artificial intelligence (AI)–driven mental health chatbots are increasingly integrated into DMHIs to address the growing demand for psychological support. These conversational tools utilize natural language processing and AI algorithms to simulate human interactions, offering personalized support for various mental health issues, particularly depression and anxiety. This chapter highlights how AI-driven mental health apps incorporate therapeutic conditions essential for user engagement and effectiveness. We systematically review and synthesize evidence from user-focused DMHI studies published in the last decade. Findings show that empathy—the pivot of therapeutic relationship in traditional counseling or psychotherapy—has been incorporated into digital interfaces such as chatbots and AI platforms through innovative features such as human-like interactions, personalized messages, reassurance, and adaptive responses that validate user emotions. A nonjudgmental space was also provided *via* anonymous interfaces, reducing fears of stigma by using nonstigmatizing language, and allowing users to express vulnerability more openly than in traditional settings. Unconditional positive regard was provided through consistent supportive language, active listening cues, and design elements that encourage trust and loyalty. Digital mental health tools are a promising solution for people dealing with mild to moderate mental health challenges, such as anxiety or stress, or for those who face barriers to traditional therapy, such as

**Corresponding author*: joeythangal@pondiuni.ac.in

Raghavendra M. Devadas, Vani Hiremani, Preethi, Praveen Gujjar, Sapna R. and Manoj Shettar (eds.) Psychiatry and Technology, (115–160) © 2026 Scrivener Publishing LLC

cost or location. They provide easy access and are available anytime, anywhere, along with personalized support tailored to individual needs and structured help through evidence-based techniques.

Keywords: Digital mental health interventions, chatbots, mental health apps, AI-based therapy

5.1 Introduction

The National Mental Health Survey of India estimates that 7.39% of individuals between the ages of 18 and 29 years experience mental disorders, excluding tobacco use disorders [1]. However, help-seeking and access to treatment remain significantly low due to an array of individual, institutional, and logistical barriers. India has only 0.7 mental health professionals per 100,000 people, glaringly below the recommended minimum of three psychiatrists per 100,000 population [2]. The treatment gap is 73.6% for severe mental disorders, 85% for common mental disorders, and 91.1% for substance use disorders [1].

The COVID-19 pandemic has worsened mental health issues globally. Studies have shown increased levels of depression, anxiety, and stress during lockdowns, with students and healthcare professionals being most affected [3]. The shortage of mental health professionals in low- and middle-income countries, including India, has been a long-standing issue [4]. This shortage is particularly concerning, given the increased mental health burden during the recent pandemic [5]. Frontline healthcare workers are especially vulnerable to mental health problems, experiencing anxiety, depression, burnout, and insomnia. Experts recommend effective communication, administrative support, mental health screening and interventions, and measures to reduce stigma and misinformation [6] to counter the challenges posed by the mounting mental health problems in the country. Expansion of mental health infrastructure and scaling up of mental health professionals are inevitable in addressing India's mental health services deficit. Harnessing the potential of digital technologies can help bridge the supply–demand gap and mitigate the problem. This chapter explores how traditional therapeutic interventions are provided using digital platforms under the broader rubric of digital mental health interventions (DMHIs). More specifically, we examine how the three core Rogerian conditions for an effective therapeutic alliance between the client and the therapist are incorporated into DMHIs. We analyze the experiences of clients who use chatbots for mental health support and identify factors that enhance their effectiveness. In the end, we discuss the shortcomings of DMHIs and suggest measures for their improvement.

5.1.1 Digital Mental Health Interventions

DMHIs are technology-driven approaches such as smartphone applications, web-based programs, virtual reality, wearable devices, and video games that are utilized in the field of mental health for promotion, prevention, education, assessment, and treatment [7, 8]. Smartphone applications are text-based messaging interfaces facilitated by human coaches or artificial intelligence (AI)–driven chatbots. AI-driven mental health chatbots are increasingly integrated into DMHIs to address the growing demand for psychological support [9]. The AI chatbot Wysa offers personalized emotional support through text-based conversations [10]. Another such chatbot, Tess, provides an array of modules that users can select according to their specific needs. For example, the module on Cognitive Distortions helps users identify and challenge maladaptive thought patterns. Other modules focus on stress management, mindfulness, and emotion regulation [11].

Studies have shown promising results in reducing psychological distress among AI chatbot users when compared to inactive control groups [12]. A meta-analysis on randomized controlled trials has indicated the efficacy of smartphone-based psychological interventions in reducing anxiety [13], suggesting that digital mental health apps can be effective therapeutic tools. Chatbots also provide advantages such as accessibility, cost-effectiveness, and early detection of mental health problems [14]. These conversational tools utilize natural language processing and AI algorithms to simulate human interactions, offering personalized support for various mental health issues, particularly depression and anxiety.

5.1.2 Therapeutic Conditions in Mental Health Apps

A secure therapeutic alliance between a client and therapist is one of the most important factors for a successful outcome. The therapeutic relationship in modern psychotherapy and counseling has evolved throughout the 20th century. Carl Rogers identified three core conditions essential for a successful therapeutic environment: empathy, unconditional positive regard, and congruence [16]. Hence, to establish a strong therapeutic connection between users and the chatbots, these core Rogerian principles must be incorporated into the app. It remains unknown how, and to what extent, digital mental health apps establish a therapeutic alliance with users [15]. This chapter seeks to throw light on this question by examining how AI-driven mental health apps incorporate therapeutic conditions essential for user engagement and effectiveness. We review and synthesize evidence from user-focused DMHI studies published in the last decade.

5.2 Methods

A comprehensive literature search was conducted across PubMed, ScienceDirect, Scopus, Google Scholar, and the *Journal of Medical Internet Research* for relevant articles published from 2015 to 2024. The keywords used to search relevant articles were "digital mental health," "eMental health," "mental health apps," "therapeutic conditions," "therapeutic alliance," "unconditional positive regard," "empathy," and "congruence." The search also included combinations of these keywords using the Boolean operators "AND" and "OR." The initial search retrieved a total of 216 studies. After removing studies published in languages other than English and duplications, 133 studies were retained. Further screening excluded 17 review articles and 92 studies that did not align with the study's objectives. Articles were excluded primarily due to their focus on practitioner perspectives rather than user experiences, lack of full-text availability, or misalignment with the evaluation of DMHIs. Finally, 24 studies were retained for the analysis. The studies include randomized clinical trials, qualitative interviews, and direct textual analyses assessing the effectiveness of DMHIs based on user experiences.

We included studies that:

- were published between 2015 and 2024 in English.
- had full-text availability.
- assessed the effectiveness of DMHIs based on user experiences.
- used randomized clinical trials, qualitative interviews, or direct textual analysis of user responses.
- focused solely on user experiences, excluding practitioner perspectives or views.
- evaluated interventions delivered *via* apps or digital platforms.

We excluded studies that:

- were unpublished manuscripts, commentary pieces, opinion articles, or reviews.
- focused on practitioner experiences rather than user experiences.
- did not provide extractable outcome data.

All abstracts from the database search were independently evaluated based on the inclusion and exclusion criteria by the first author. Later, the chosen articles were independently verified by the second author. The full texts of selected papers were retrieved for an independent assessment, and relevant data were extracted. A summary of the studies has been provided in Table 5.1 (Appendix 1). The extracted data were checked for accuracy and completeness. Data extracted included the authors and year, study design, number of samples, the apps used in the study, and the intervention adopted.

A systematic narrative method was conducted to synthesize the studies.

5.3 Results and Discussion

The studies on DMHIs encompassed a variety of methodological approaches, each offering unique insights into their effectiveness and user experiences. There were 10 randomized clinical trials [17–26], typically involving experimental designs with control and intervention groups to assess efficacy, often measuring outcomes such as symptom reduction or engagement over time. Four single-arm studies [27–30] utilized uncontrolled designs to explore feasibility and acceptability in a single group, focusing on preliminary outcomes without a comparison group. Three mixed-methods studies [31–33] combined quantitative data, such as symptom scores or usage statistics, with qualitative insights from user feedback to provide a comprehensive view of both measurable effects and subjective experiences. Five qualitative studies [12, 34–37] used interviews or thematic analyses to delve deeply into user perceptions, identifying themes such as therapeutic alliance or usability challenges. Lastly, two observational pre–post studies [38, 39] assessed changes in outcomes, such as anxiety or suicidal ideation, before and after intervention without randomization, relying on large-scale user data to infer effectiveness. Together, these diverse methods highlight the multifaceted evaluation of digital mental health tools across efficacy, user satisfaction, and practical implementation.

Several studies focused on young adults and adolescents (16–25 years) who experienced moderate to severe mental health issues [36] and adolescents (12–18 years) recovering from concussions. Others, such as He *et al.* [19] and Karkosz *et al.* [21], examined young adults with depressive and anxiety symptoms in subclinical ranges. Adults with specific conditions, including individuals with chronic pain [23, 33], postpartum depression [25, 37], and suicidal ideation [39] were also studied. Studies such as those of Beatty *et al.* [31] and Darcy *et al.* [38] included large samples with anxiety and depression, ranging from subclinical to diagnosed cases, whereas Brotherdale *et al.* [34] targeted a smaller group with severe diagnoses such as schizophrenia and bipolar disorder. Sample sizes varied widely, from small qualitative cohorts (e.g., n = 10) [36] to massive observational datasets (e.g., n = 152,783 interactions) [32].

5.3.1 Features of the Digital Mental Health Apps

The DMHIs evaluated across these studies (see Table 5.2 [Appendix 2]) encompass a wide array of applications designed to address diverse psychological needs and conditions. Apps such as Headspace, Calm, and Insight Timer are frequently used for meditation and relaxation, helping users manage anxiety, improve sleep, and enhance overall well-being. Apps such as Wysa, used across multiple studies [31, 33, 35], serve functions such as mood tracking, anxiety management, and chronic pain support through interactions rooted in cognitive behavioral therapy (CBT). Other apps, such as MOST+ [27], provide web-based counseling and peer support for severe mental health conditions, whereas MYLO [12] facilitates reflective conversations using the Method of Levels therapy. Apps for populations with specific needs such as MomMoodBooster [37] for perinatal depression and the Meru Health Program [39] for suicidal ideation were also catered to by integrating therapist support with digital modules. Additionally, apps such as Fido [21] and XiaoE [19] focused on subclinical symptoms with CBT-based chatbots, whereas tools such as Pixel and Habit Tracking [34] emphasized journaling and behavior tracking to identify mood patterns and reinforce positive habits. This diversity highlights the adaptability of digital tools, ranging from general wellness (e.g., Smiling Mind) to targeted therapeutic interventions (e.g., ERICA for emotion regulation), catering to varied user feedback and mental health goals.

5.3.2 Motivational Factors behind Using Mental Health Apps

Users turn to DMHIs for a variety of reasons as shown in Figure 5.1, ranging from personal interest to external recommendations.

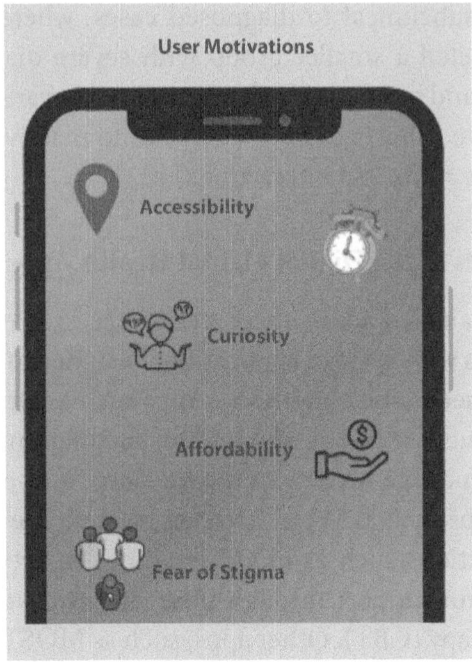

Figure 5.1 Motivational factors in mental health app usage.

Some individuals use these apps as an additional aid upon the recommendation of mental health professionals, whereas others turn to them due to the unavailability of traditional services or difficulty communicating with people. Marketing strategies, such as targeted advertisements, also play a role in drawing users to these platforms [34]. Additionally, users report engaging with DMHIs for specific functions such as mood tracking, symptom management, and developing therapeutic skills. Some were intrigued by the way chatbots function and explored these tools out of curiosity. The barriers to traditional mental healthcare, such as fear of stigma, confidentiality concerns, poor mental health literacy, and financial constraints, further drive individuals toward digital alternatives. Many also prefer DMHIs due to social isolation or geographical distance, making these tools a more accessible option when in-person therapy is not feasible [27].

5.3.3 Effectiveness of DMHIs

The effectiveness of DMHIs refers to the degree to which that intervention successfully produces a desired result. This review examined 24 studies that analyzed 37 different mental health apps. In the studies, the key indicators of the effectiveness of the DMHIs were the degree of engagement, time spent on the application, and users' ratings and feedback and through quantitative questionnaires such as the Patient Health Questionnaire-9. Additionally, effectiveness was also assessed through clinical outcomes such as symptom reduction or long-term user adherence.

As shown in Figure 5.2, out of the 37 apps, 18 (49%) were found to be helpful, leading to significant improvements in symptoms such as anxiety, depression, stress, and mood regulation. However, six apps (16%) were not effective, and four (11%) showed mixed results. The remaining nine (24%) lacked clear evidence, often because the studies focused on exploring the apps rather than measuring their impact. Encouragingly, 21 of the 24 studies reported that the apps helped reduce mental health symptoms, with improvements in anxiety reduction, mood regulation, and emotional well-being being the most common benefits.

The apps can be categorized into five groups: meditation and mindfulness (7 apps), CBT and psychoeducation (11 apps), mood

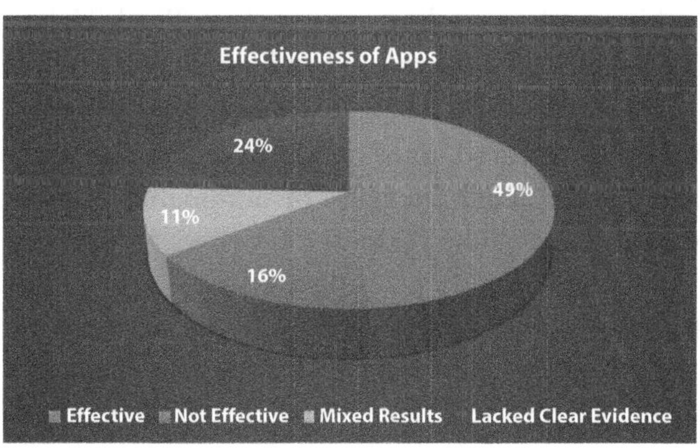

Figure 5.2 Effectiveness of mental health apps.

tracking and journaling (5 apps), self-help (8 apps), and chatbot-based interventions (6 apps). We discuss the effectiveness of each app below.

Meditation and mindfulness apps

Headspace, Calm, Balance, and Smiling Mind were effective among the meditation and mindfulness apps. Users liked the structured meditation programs, personalization options, and engagement tools such as reminders and progress tracking. In contrast, Abide, Insight Timer, and Tomo received mixed reviews. These apps lacked structured programs and interactive features, suggesting that user engagement depends on both content quality and how it is delivered.

CBT and psychoeducation apps

Clear Fear, Calm Harm, Life Flex, Spark, CBASPath, and a 4-week mindfulness-based program [36] performed well for CBT and psychoeducation apps. These apps use well-established therapeutic techniques and interactive features tailored to specific symptoms. On the other hand, the Insight App, Woebot, XiaoE, MomMoodBooster, and myCompass were less effective. Many users felt these apps did not provide enough real-time therapist interaction, emphasizing the need for human support alongside digital tools.

Mood tracking and journaling apps

Mood tracking and journaling apps such as Pixel, Habit Tracking, and Today I Am were effective. They helped users reflect on their emotions and behaviors through simple, goal-oriented designs. However, Health Assured and For Me were less successful because they lacked personalized feedback or actionable insights, making them feel more passive than helpful.

Self-help apps

Self-help apps such as Brain In Hand, Self-Help for Anxiety Management, I Am Sober, and Meru Health Program performed well. Their success was linked to immediate support, useful strategies, community features, and therapist-assisted elements. In contrast,

MYLO, MOST+, the Internet-Based Routine Process Monitoring and Feedback System, and Fido did not perform as well. They relied too much on self-guided approaches without enough personalization or real-time support, suggesting that hybrid models (combining human and digital support) may be more effective than fully automated interventions.

Chatbot-based apps

Chatbot-based apps such as Wysa, ERICA, and Koko were effective because they provided meaningful conversations, cognitive restructuring tools, and emotional support. However, Woebot, SimSimi, and XiaoE were less effective due to their lack of personalization, structure, and engagement features. This highlights the need for well-designed, engaging AI-driven tools to maintain user interest and effectiveness.

Individual differences in interaction and engagement with digital interventions are a scope for further studies. These differences might include age, technological familiarity, or the severity of mental health conditions, which could influence how users interact with and benefit from these tools [40]. The findings show that although these digital tools hold promise, their effectiveness varies.

5.3.4 The Therapeutic Relationship in DMHIs

The therapeutic relationship, or the therapeutic alliance, has long been a key factor in successful mental health interventions. Traditionally, this bond is built through direct human interaction. However, with the rise of DMHIs, researchers have explored how this relationship can be adapted to digital platforms. Seven studies [12, 17, 18, 27, 28, 34, 38] reveal both opportunities and challenges in fostering a meaningful connection between users and digital mental health tools. These studies show a wide range of user experiences, from perceiving apps as supportive companions to seeing them as impersonal tools. They also highlight how digital platforms can reflect core aspects of Carl Rogers' therapeutic conditions, empathy, unconditional positive regard, and congruence, while introducing new dimensions such as accessibility and autonomy [22, 24, 31, 38].

Brotherdale *et al.* [34] categorize users' connections with DMHIs into three types: personification, passive connection, and nonhuman perception. Some users develop a strong emotional bond with these tools, particularly those who live alone or have limited social interactions. They view these apps as loyal companions, similar to how Rogers emphasized empathy and unconditional positive regard in therapy. Features such as human-like voices and interactive elements, such as community engagement tools [36], enhance this feeling of being understood. Others form a more functional relationship with these tools, using them primarily for structured check-ins or emotional offloading rather than emotional connection. However, individuals with prior therapy experience often find these apps lacking nuanced empathy, making the digital experience feel less authentic and disrupting the sense of congruence that Rogers deemed essential [22].

One major advantage of digital mental health tools is their accessibility. As noted by Brotherdale *et al.* [34] and Andrews *et al.* [18], user-friendly designs, personalized features, and 24/7 availability help users feel supported on their terms [23, 29, 35]. This aligns with Rogers' principles by ensuring users feel heard and cared for in a way that fits their lifestyle. Alvarez-Jimenez *et al.* [27] highlight how peer and clinician interactions within platforms such as MOST+ can enhance social connectedness and well-being, similar to how empathy is fostered in traditional therapy. Woebot's empathetic language and personalized responses can create a sense of connection, even when users fully know they are interacting with AI [38].

Empowerment and choice also play a critical role in the digital therapeutic alliance. As Brotherdale *et al.* [34] point out, allowing users to engage with these tools at their own pace reflects Rogers' client-centered approach. For some, this autonomy enhances a sense of control and strengthens the alliance. However, too many choices can feel overwhelming for individuals with more severe symptoms, highlighting the need for balanced guidance. Rather than deep therapeutic engagement, many see these tools as safe spaces for self-reflection [12, 21, 33].

The idea of digital platforms as "safe spaces" is particularly valuable. Brotherdale *et al.* [34] describe how these apps provide a judgment-free environment where users feel comfortable expressing their thoughts. This is especially meaningful for minority groups or individuals concerned about stigma. These tools reinforce the therapeutic alliance by offering a secure and confidential space. Amo *et al.* [17], He *et al.* [19], and Forman-Hoffman *et al.* [28] also highlighted how interactive, evidence-based features, such as CBT techniques, help sustain engagement across different populations, including those in marginalized communities. This emulates the Rogerian principle of empathy by enabling customized support systems in a nonjudgmental environment.

5.3.5 Effectiveness Enhancing and Inhibiting Features of the DMHIs

Effective DMHIs tend to share features such as personalization, structured content, and hybrid support models that blend digital tools with human interaction (Figure 5.3). Conversely, as shown in Figure 5.4, apps that lack engagement, interactivity, or tailored

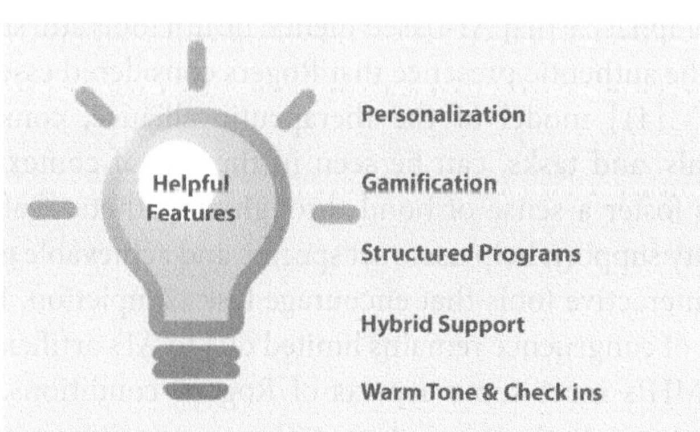

Figure 5.3 Features that augmented the effectiveness of the apps.

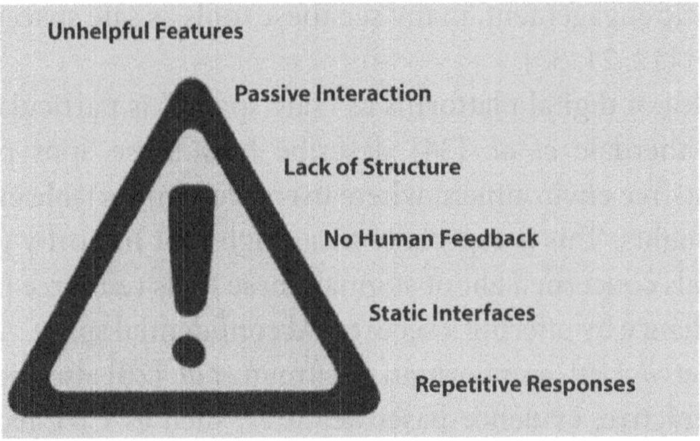

Figure 5.4 Features of the apps that attenuated the effectiveness of the apps.

approaches often fell short, underscoring the importance of designing interventions that meet diverse user needs.

Despite these benefits, challenges remain. Gaffney *et al.* [12] note that overly repetitive or robotic responses can weaken the alliance, making interactions feel less human. Similarly, Morris *et al.* [22] suggest that AI struggles to replicate the depth of human empathy, with many users preferring peer-driven support over automated responses. Andrews *et al.* [18] highlighted that engagement tends to drop when these tools lack a stepped-care approach, suggesting that whereas self-guided interventions align with autonomy, therapist-assisted models may better sustain the therapeutic connection. These findings emphasize that AI-based mental health tools still struggle to embody the authentic presence that Rogers considered essential.

Bordin's [41] model of the therapeutic alliance, consisting of bond, goals, and tasks, can be seen in the digital context. Digital platforms foster a sense of bond through empathetic features and community support, help users set specific and achievable goals, and provide interactive tools that encourage task completion. However, the depth of congruence remains limited due to AI's artificial nature. While DMHIs meet some aspects of Rogers' conditions, offering validation (empathy), a nonjudgmental space (positive regard), and transparency (such as Woebot openly identifying as a bot), they are best suited as supplementary tools rather than full replacements for human therapy. They appear most effective for individuals with mild to moderate symptoms, where self-awareness and engagement are already relatively strong [27, 34].

Overall, although DMHIs can support and enhance the therapeutic alliance in meaningful ways, they cannot yet fully replicate the depth of human connection found in traditional therapy. Their strength lies in accessibility, autonomy, and structured support, making them valuable for individuals seeking self-guided mental healthcare or additional reinforcement between therapy sessions. However, for deeper therapeutic needs, human interaction remains irreplaceable.

5.4 Conclusion

We found that *empathy*—the pivot of therapeutic relationship in traditional counseling or psychotherapy—had been incorporated into the digital interfaces such as chatbots and AI platforms by their developers through innovative features such as human-like interactions, personalized messages, reassurance, and adaptive responses that validate user emotions. A nonjudgmental space was also provided *via* anonymous interfaces, reducing fears of stigma by using nonstigmatizing language, and allowing users to express vulnerability more openly than in traditional settings. Unconditional positive regard is provided through consistent supportive language, active listening cues, and design elements that encourage trust and loyalty.

We also identified factors that enhance DMHI effectiveness. They include (i) personalization—customizable interfaces, goal-setting features, and user-specific recommendations that increase engagement and perceived empathy; (ii) accessibility—immediate, on-demand support, and asynchronous interaction that allow users to seek help conveniently; (iii) autonomy and empowerment—options for activities, strategies, and pacing that foster user control and adherence; (iv) cultural sensitivity—tailored content that respects cultural differences to improve emotional resonance and user satisfaction; (v) trustworthiness—consistent use of validating statements and active listening cues that build loyalty and a sense of connection; (vi) evidence-based branding—highlighting the use of established therapeutic methods (e.g., CBT) and evidence-based practices that enhance credibility, increase user trust, and boost engagement. On the other hand, barriers to effectiveness include unrealistic user expectations, lack of nuanced feedback compared to human therapists, user skepticism toward technology, and poor integration with offline support.

In conclusion, our paper highlights how DMHIs demonstrate the potential to replicate key aspects of the therapeutic alliance, making them effective tools for mental health support. Enhancing empathy, personalization, and cultural sensitivity while addressing user-specific needs can further bolster their effectiveness. By integrating these principles, developers can design interventions that align with Rogerian conditions and improve mental health outcomes and overall retention rate. Digital mental health tools are a promising solution for people dealing with mild to moderate mental health challenges, such as anxiety or stress, or for those who face barriers to traditional therapy, such as cost or location. They provide easy access and are available anytime, anywhere, along with personalized support tailored to individual needs and structured help through evidence-based techniques. For example, apps such as Headspace and Wysa have been shown to reduce symptoms of depression and anxiety, offering user convenience and a sense of control.

5.5 Limitations and Future Directions

However, these tools have limitations. They cannot fully replace the deep connection and empathy that come from human therapists, which is especially important for more severe mental health conditions. Research highlights that DMHIs work better when they include some human support, such as guidance from a therapist, rather than being entirely self-guided. Their effectiveness also depends on factors such as the user's tech skills, cultural background, and the seriousness of their condition.

Rather than standing alone, DMHIs are most valuable as complementary to traditional care. Technological advancements could make these tools even more effective, but human interaction will remain essential for addressing complex emotional needs. The true strength of DMHIs lies in expanding access to mental health support, especially for those who might otherwise go without help. To maximize their impact, we should focus on blending digital tools with human-led care, creating a practical and compassionate balance.

Acknowledgments

The authors express their gratitude to the editorial team and the anonymous peer reviewers who provided constructive feedback and valuable suggestions that immensely contributed to the improvement of this chapter.

AI disclosure statement: The author acknowledges the use of AI-based tools for minor language editing or grammatical correction. However, all intellectual contributions, analyses, and conclusions presented in this chapter are entirely the author's own.

References

1. Chadda, R.K., Youth & mental health: Challenges ahead. *Indian J. Med. Res.*, 148, 4, 359–361, Oct. 2018, doi: 10.4103/ijmr.IJMR_1585_18.
2. Jha, D.N., India needs 3 psychiatrists per lakh population, has only 0.7, 2023.
3. Rehman, U., *et al.*, Depression, Anxiety and Stress Among Indians in Times of Covid-19 Lockdown. *Community Ment. Health J.*, 57, 1, 42–48, Jan. 2021, doi: 10.1007/s10597-020-00664-x.
4. Bruckner, T.A., *et al.*, The mental health workforce gap in low- and middle-income countries: A needs-based approach. *Bull. World Health Organ.*, 89, 3, 184–194, Mar. 2011, doi: 10.2471/BLT.10.082784.
5. Tiwari, V., L.R., S.A., B.S., Mental health disorders during COVID-19 pandemic: A review. *J. Pharm. Res. Int.*, 33, 64A, 59–65, 2021.

6. Gupta, S. and Sahoo, S., Pandemic and mental health of the frontline healthcare workers: a review and implications in the Indian context amidst COVID-19, Oct. 01, 2020, BMJ Publishing Group. doi: 10.1136/gpsych-2020-100284.
7. Khanna, R., Robinson, N., O'Donnell, M., Eyre, H., Smith, E., Affective Computing in Psychotherapy. *Adv. Psychiatry Behav. Health*, 2, 1, 95–105, Sep. 2022, doi: 10.1016/j.ypsc.2022.05.006.
8. Kaveladze, B. and Schueller, S.M., Chapter 8 - A digital therapeutic alliance in digital mental health, in: *Digital Therapeutics for Mental Health and Addiction*, N. Jacobson, T. Kowatsch, L. Marsch (Eds.), pp. 87–98, Academic Press, Amsterdam, 2023, doi: 10.1016/B978-0-323-90045-4.00009-5.
9. Boucher, E.M., *et al.*, Artificially intelligent chatbots in digital mental health interventions: a review. *Expert Rev. Med. Devices*, 18, sup1, 37–49, Dec. 2021, doi: 10.1080/17434440.2021.2013200.
10. Inkster, B., Sarda, S., Subramanian, V., An Empathy-Driven, Conversational Artificial Intelligence Agent (Wysa) for Digital Mental Well-Being: Real-World Data Evaluation Mixed-Methods Study. *JMIR Mhealth Uhealth*, 6, 11, e12106, Nov. 2018, doi: 10.2196/12106.
11. Dosovitsky, G., Pineda, B.S., Jacobson, N.C., Chang, C., Bunge, E.L., Artificial Intelligence Chatbot for Depression: Descriptive Study of Usage (Preprint), Nov. 2019, doi: 10.2196/preprints.17065.
12. Gaffney, H., Mansell, W., Tai, S., Agents of change: Understanding the therapeutic processes associated with the helpfulness of therapy for mental health problems with relational agent MYLO. *Digital Health*, 6, 2055207620911580, Jan. 2020, doi: 10.1177/2055207620911580.
13. Firth, J., Torous, J., Nicholas, J., Carney, R., Rosenbaum, S., Sarris, J., Can smartphone mental health interventions reduce symptoms of anxiety? A meta-analysis of randomized controlled trials. *J. Affect. Disord.*, 218, 15–22, Aug. 2017, doi: 10.1016/j.jad.2017.04.046.
14. Lopes, R.M., Silva, A.F., Rodrigues, A.C.A., Melo, V., Chatbots for Well-Being: Exploring the Impact of Artificial Intelligence on Mood Enhancement and Mental Health. *Eur. Psychiatry*, 67, S1, S550–S551, Apr. 2024, doi: 10.1192/j.eurpsy.2024.1143.
15. D'Alfonso, S., Lederman, R., Bucci, S., Berry, K., The Digital Therapeutic Alliance and Human-Computer Interaction. *JMIR Ment. Health*, 7, 12, Dec. 2020, doi: 10.2196/21895.

16. Witty, M.C., Client-Centered Therapy, in: *Handbook of Homework Assignments in Psychotherapy*, Kazantzis, N.and LL'Abate, L. (eds) pp. 35–50, Springer, Boston, MA, 2007. doi: 10.1007/978-0-387-29681-4_3.
17. Amo, V., Prentice, M., Lieder, F., A Gamified Mobile App That Helps People Develop the Metacognitive Skills to Cope With Stressful Situations and Difficult Emotions: Formative Assessment of the InsightApp. *JMIR Form. Res.*, 7, e44429, Jun. 2023, doi: 10.2196/44429.
18. Andrews, B., Klein, B., Van Nguyen, H., Corboy, D., McLaren, S., Watson, S., Efficacy of a Digital Mental Health Biopsychosocial Transdiagnostic Intervention With or Without Therapist Assistance for Adults With Anxiety and Depression: Adaptive Randomized Controlled Trial. *J. Med. Internet Res.*, 25, e45135, Jun. 2023, doi: 10.2196/45135.
19. He, Y., *et al.*, Mental Health Chatbot for Young Adults With Depressive Symptoms During the COVID-19 Pandemic: Single-Blind, Three-Arm Randomized Controlled Trial. *J. Med. Internet Res.*, 24, 11, e40719, Nov. 2022, doi: 10.2196/40719.
20. Hopman, K., Richards, D., Norberg, M.M., A digital coach to promote emotion regulation skills. *Multimodal Technol. Interact.*, 7, 6, 57, 2023, [Online]. Available: https://www.mdpi.com/2414-4088/7/6/57.
21. Karkosz, S., Szymański, R., Sanna, K., Michałowski, J., Effectiveness of a Web-Based and Mobile Therapy Chatbot on Anxiety and Depressive Symptoms in Subclinical Young Adults: Randomized Controlled Trial. *JMIR Form. Res.*, 8, e47960, Mar. 2024, doi: 10.2196/47960.
22. Morris, R.R., Kouddous, K., Kshirsagar, R., Schueller, S.M., Towards an Artificially Empathic Conversational Agent for Mental Health Applications: System Design and User Perceptions. *J. Med. Internet Res.*, 20, 6, e10148, Jun. 2018, doi: 10.2196/10148.
23. Sinha, C., Cheng, A.L., Kadaba, M., Adherence and Engagement With a Cognitive Behavioral Therapy–Based Conversational Agent (Wysa for Chronic Pain) Among Adults With Chronic Pain: Survival Analysis. *JMIR Form. Res.*, 6, 5, e37302, May 2022, doi: 10.2196/37302.
24. Stefana, A., Fusar-Poli, P., Vieta, E., Youngstrom, E.A., Effectiveness of a Novel Web-Based Intervention to Enhance Therapeutic Relationships and Treatment Outcomes in Adult Individual Psychotherapy: Randomized Controlled Trial and Analysis of Predictors of Dropouts. *JMIR Ment. Health*, 11, e63234, Nov. 2024, doi: 10.2196/63234.

25. Suharwardy, S., *et al.*, Feasibility and impact of a mental health chatbot on postpartum mental health: a randomized controlled trial. *AJOG Global Rep.*, 3, 3, 100165, Aug. 2023, doi: 10.1016/j.xagr.2023.100165.
26. Whitton, A.E., *et al.*, Breaking Open the Black Box: Isolating the Most Potent Features of a Web and Mobile Phone-Based Intervention for Depression, Anxiety, and Stress. *JMIR Ment. Health*, 2, 1, Jan. 2015, doi: 10.2196/mental.3573.
27. Alvarez-Jimenez, M., *et al.*, A Novel Multimodal Digital Service (Moderated Online Social Therapy+) for Help-Seeking Young People Experiencing Mental Ill-Health: Pilot Evaluation Within a National Youth E-Mental Health Service. *J. Med. Internet Res.*, 22, 8, e17155, Aug. 2020, doi: 10.2196/17155.
28. Forman-Hoffman, V.L., *et al.*, Engagement, Satisfaction, and Mental Health Outcomes Across Different Residential Subgroup Users of a Digital Mental Health Relational Agent: Exploratory Single-Arm Study. *JMIR Form. Res.*, 7, e46473, Sep. 2023, doi: 10.2196/46473.
29. Miller, I., *et al.*, Self-Guided Digital Intervention for Depression in Adolescents: Feasibility and Preliminary Efficacy Study. *JMIR Form. Res.*, 7, e43260, Nov. 2023, doi: 10.2196/43260.
30. Netter, A.-L., Beintner, I., Brakemeier, E.-L., Adding an App-Based Intervention to the Cognitive Behavioral Analysis System of Psychotherapy in Routine Outpatient Psychotherapy Treatment: Proof-of-Concept Study. *JMIR Form. Res.*, 6, 8, e35482, Aug. 2022, doi: 10.2196/35482.
31. Beatty, C., Malik, T., Meheli, S., Sinha, C., Evaluating the Therapeutic Alliance With a Free-Text CBT Conversational Agent (Wysa): A Mixed-Methods Study. *Front. Digital Health*, 4, Apr. 2022, doi: 10.3389/fdgth.2022.847991.
32. Chin, H., *et al.*, The Potential of Chatbots for Emotional Support and Promoting Mental Well-Being in Different Cultures: Mixed Methods Study. *J. Med. Internet Res.*, 25, e51712, Oct. 2023, doi: 10.2196/51712.
33. Meheli, S., Sinha, C., Kadaba, M., Understanding People With Chronic Pain Who Use a Cognitive Behavioral Therapy–Based Artificial Intelligence Mental Health App (Wysa): Mixed Methods Retrospective Observational Study. *JMIR Hum. Factors*, 9, 2, e35671, Apr. 2022, doi: 10.2196/35671.

34. Brotherdale, R., Berry, K., Bucci, S., A qualitative study exploring the digital therapeutic alliance with fully automated smartphone apps. *Digital Health*, 10, Jan. 2024, doi: 10.1177/20552076241277712.
35. Malik, T., Ambrose, A.J., Sinha, C., Evaluating User Feedback for an Artificial Intelligence–Enabled, Cognitive Behavioral Therapy–Based Mental Health App (Wysa): Qualitative Thematic Analysis. *JMIR Hum. Factors*, 9, 2, e35668, Apr. 2022, doi: 10.2196/35668.
36. O'Kane, K.M.K., *et al.*, Development of Therapeutic Alliance and Social Presence in a Digital Intervention for Pediatric Concussion: Qualitative Exploratory Study. *JMIR Form. Res.*, 8, e49133, Mar. 2024, doi: 10.2196/49133.
37. Solness, C.L., Holdefer, P.J., Hsu, T., Thomas, E.B.K., O'Hara, M.W., Relationship Factors in Internet-Delivered Psychological Interventions for Veterans Experiencing Postpartum Depression: Qualitative Analysis. *JMIR Ment. Health*, 10, e46061, Aug. 2023, doi: 10.2196/46061.
38. Darcy, A., Daniels, J., Salinger, D., Wicks, P., Robinson, A., Evidence of Human-Level Bonds Established With a Digital Conversational Agent: Cross-Sectional, Retrospective Observational Study. *JMIR Form. Res.*, 5, 5, e27868, May 2021, doi: 10.2196/27868.
39. Nelson, B.W., Forman-Hoffman, V.L., Peiper, N.C., Preliminary Effectiveness of a Therapist-Supported Digital Mental Health Intervention in Reducing Suicidal Ideation. *Arch. Suicide Res.*, 28, 3, 934–947, Jul. 2024, doi: 10.1080/13811118.2023.2262540.
40. Garrido, S., *et al.*, What Works and What Doesn't Work? A Systematic Review of Digital Mental Health Interventions for Depression and Anxiety in Young People. *Front. Psychiatry*, 10, Nov. 2019, doi: 10.3389/fpsyt.2019.00759.
41. Bordin, E.S., The generalizability of the psychoanalytic concept of the working alliance. *Psychother. Theory Res. Pract.*, 16, 3, 252–260, 1979, doi: 10.1037/h0085885.

Appendix 1

Table 5.1 Characteristics of the studies included in the systematic review.

Sl. no.	Study	Method	Conditions	Major findings
1	[27]	Pilot evaluation Uncontrolled single-group study n = 93 Age: 16–25 y	Moderate to severe mental health conditions (e.g., psychological distress, depression, loneliness). Addresses multiple issues.	MOST+ was feasible, acceptable, and safe; 98% had a positive experience, 82% felt better, and 92% would recommend it. Significant improvements in psychological distress, perceived stress, depression, loneliness, social support, autonomy, and self-competence. The inclusion of support groups with individuals facing similar conditions enhances the experience by fostering a sense of community and peer support. No serious adverse events.
2	[17]	Two experiments: Experiment 1 (n = 63) (single session), Experiment 2 (n = 142) (2-wk randomized controlled trial)	Stress and emotion regulation	A single session with the app helped reduce emotional distress and unhelpful thoughts while promoting more positive thinking and actions. These effects were confirmed with repeated use. Lasting impact: Benefits lasted for at least 2 wk Features such as self-reflection prompts, example answers, and rating scales were advantageous. The app effectively tracked changes in metacognitive skills and mental health, making it a valuable research tool. Users reported increased self-awareness and improved coping mechanisms. Gamified UI-enhanced engagement, motivation, and skill development.

(Continued)

Table 5.1 Characteristics of the studies included in the systematic review. (*Continued*)

Sl. no.	Study	Method	Conditions	Major findings
3	[18]	Randomized adaptive clinical trial with assessments at Weeks 0, 3, 6, 9, and 21 n = 103	Subclinical symptoms of anxiety and depression	Both conditions (with and without therapist assistance) showed a significant reduction in symptoms of anxiety and depression. The app includes cognitive behavioral therapy (CBT) techniques to help users manage their thoughts and behaviors, neuroplasticity principles, and brain training to improve brain flexibility and adaptability. Self-guided structure helps them to move at their own pace and comfort. By the 3-mo follow-up, ~69% of participants no longer met diagnostic criteria for anxiety or depression. Results show high attrition and low completion rates in the absence of stepped care.
4	[31]	Mixed-methods study Quantitative analysis (N = 1205) Qualitative analysis (N = 212)	Anxiety and depression symptoms	Users developed a therapeutic alliance with Wysa. Content analysis revealed users expressed gratitude, personified the chatbot, and acknowledged a relational bond. Helpful features: Use of evidence-based CBT, ACT, and positive psychology techniques, free-text conversational AI allows natural interactions, Anonymity and privacy. Unhelpful: AI misunderstandings and irrelevant responses led to user frustration, perceived limitations in conversational depth and complexity. Some users found the therapeutic alliance weaker than in human-led therapy.

(*Continued*)

Table 5.1 Characteristics of the studies included in the systematic review. (*Continued*)

Sl. no.	Study	Method	Conditions	Major findings
5	[34]	Qualitative semistructured interview n = 17 (current users or had used recently) RQ: What constitutes a digital therapeutic alliance	13/17 were diagnosed with depression, anxiety, personality disorders, schizophrenia, bipolar, PTSD, and OCD.	Five themes: 1: Connection: Personification (human-like bond, friendship, loyalty), passive connection (useful features, regular check-ins, human-voice elements, community presence), and nonhuman perception (lack of empathy, AI limitations). 2: Accessibility: user-friendliness (easy navigation, customization, animations) and availability (on-demand support, crisis accessibility, nighttime assistance). 3: Choice and empowerment: Facilitated by control (decision-making flexibility, autonomy) and accountability. 4: Goals and expectations: Shaped by differing purposes (short-term symptom management) and lower expectations (outlet for expression, reduced reliance on apps' responses). 5: Safe space: lack of judgment (reduced stigma, anonymity) and loyalty/reliance (predictability, confidentiality, no false promises, reduced burden on others).

(*Continued*)

Table 5.1 Characteristics of the studies included in the systematic review. (*Continued*)

Sl. no.	Study	Method	Conditions	Major findings
6	[32]	Mixed-methods study N = 152,783 user interactions (not no. of participants)	Depressive symptoms	Cultural Differences: Eastern users expressed stronger emotional intensity. Eastern users used more words related to sadness and expressed emotional vulnerability in greater detail, whereas Western users discussed broader life issues such as social and physical health more openly. Users were more open to discussing depressive moods with chatbots (49.83%) than on social media (7.53%). Helpful features: Anonymity (nonjudgmental space), and accessibility (act as virtual friends to alleviate loneliness or stress). Depressive moods were more frequently expressed later in the day, with Eastern users showing a higher frequency from late night to dawn compared to Western users.

(*Continued*)

Table 5.1 Characteristics of the studies included in the systematic review. (*Continued*)

Sl. no.	Study	Method	Conditions	Major findings
7	[38]	Cross-sectional observational study N = 100,009: registered during Nov 2019 to Apr 2020 N = 77203: registered during Jul 2020 to Aug 2020.	Anxiety and Depression	Woebot's empathetic statements, positive reinforcement, mood tracking, and personalized follow-ups contributed to user engagement and motivation. Users reported a strong working alliance with Woebot. They felt cared for and supported. Users with and without depression symptoms reported indicating that Woebot was effective for different groups. Explicitly presented as a robot: Woebot frequently reminded users that it was an AI, not a real person. This enhanced the transparency and helped manage user expectations and avoid the "uncanny valley" effect. Did not try to mimic human therapists, but rather presented as an artificial system. Explicitly mentioned how it is different from humans. Did not simulate deep emotions, instead used humor, casual language, and a friendly tone.
8	[28]	Exploratory single-arm study N = 255	Depressive and anxiety symptoms, stress, resilience, and burnout	Relational agents improved satisfaction and mental health outcomes. Users who engaged more frequently reported stronger emotional bonds and better therapeutic relationships.

(*Continued*)

Table 5.1 Characteristics of the studies included in the systematic review. (*Continued*)

Sl. no.	Study	Method	Conditions	Major findings
9	[12]	Questionnaires were completed at baseline and follow-up and qualitative interviews were conducted at follow-up N = 15 Used MYLO for 2 wk	Addresses multiple issues such as anxiety, social anxiety, depression, loneliness, bereavement, low self-esteem, concerns about work, worry, sleep problems, relationship problems, financial concerns, and career problems.	The MYLO agent fostered a therapeutic relationship leading to improved mental health. Personalized interactions and memory retention features enhanced the sense of being understood. Open-ended and nondirective questions allowed them to express themselves freely. This feature helped in enhanced self-reflection. Users find features such as a human-like tone, conversational, and validating statements, acknowledging progress, helpful and effective. Users find several unhelpful features such as repetition, confusing wording, and inappropriate responses (less cohesive responses). Some users felt the app lacked human-like abilities which hindered their engagement with the app.

(*Continued*)

Table 5.1 Characteristics of the studies included in the systematic review. (*Continued*)

Sl. no.	Study	Method	Conditions	Major findings
10	[19]	Three-arm RCT (N = 148)	Young adults with depressive symptoms	Mental health chatbots were effective in alleviating depression symptoms during the COVID-19 pandemic. AI-driven structured sessions helped reduce symptoms of depression and anxiety. Structured CBT-based interventions, such as modules for challenging cognitive distortions, improving self-esteem, relaxation exercises, and journaling, helped users with depressive symptoms. Personalization Daily task reminders help users stay consistent with the intervention. Unhelpful features: Rigid and repetitive content, technological limitations, limited emotional depth, short-term impact.

(*Continued*)

Table 5.1 Characteristics of the studies included in the systematic review. (*Continued*)

Sl. no.	Study	Method	Conditions	Major findings
11	[20]	Randomized clinical trials and qualitative feedback digital coaching (N = 138)	Emotion regulation	Digital coaching facilitated better emotion regulation through structured exercises. Real-time coaching support and guided strategies led to long-term improvements. ERICA was effective in delivering emotion regulation strategies and building a therapeutic connection. One-third of participants rated their therapeutic alliance with ERICA highly (9 or 10/10), similar to ratings expected from human therapists. This suggests that ERICA was able to establish a meaningful connection with users after interacting for a short duration (<15 min). 127/138 participants planned to apply at least one of the strategies ERICA provided. A higher intention to use strategies leads to a stronger therapeutic alliance. ERICA's design and appearance were well-received. Unhelpful features: Some participants found her voice robotic.

(*Continued*)

Table 5.1 Characteristics of the studies included in the systematic review. (*Continued*)

Sl. no.	Study	Method	Conditions	Major findings
12	[21]	Randomized controlled trial N = 81	Subclinical depression and anxiety symptoms in young adults	Reduction in anxiety and depression symptoms, which remained stable after 1 mo. Users reported helpful: real-time support, personalized feedback, and behavioral tracking, time efficiency, and shorter interventions enhanced engagement and motivation. Participants who used Fido more frequently showed a greater reduction in loneliness. Younger participants reported stronger emotional bonds with Fido. A common complaint was that the chatbot often failed to recognize user intent, leading to frustrating interactions where it stated, "I don't know what you are talking about."

(*Continued*)

Table 5.1 Characteristics of the studies included in the systematic review. (*Continued*)

Sl. no.	Study	Method	Conditions	Major findings
13	[35]	Qualitative thematic analysis of feedback (n = 7929) reported on the Google Play Store	Subclinical symptoms—address multiple issues	Users valued AI-based CBT integration. Higher adherence rates were linked to the chatbot's responsiveness. Users initially doubted AI's effectiveness but found it helpful after consistent use. Helpful features: accessibility (24/7), nonjudgmental space due to anonymity, structured interventions (e.g., journaling prompts, cognitive restructuring exercises) helped users engage effectively, users valued the AI's ability to acknowledge their emotions and provide supportive responses, personalizing their experience, such as setting goals or choosing response styles, Automated responses and step-by-step guidance reduced the effort required from users, increasing engagement. Barriers: AI's responses were too generic, robotic, or repetitive, leading to disengagement, limited context awareness, lack of deeper conversation capabilities, and the ability to remember past interactions; responses were too basic.

(*Continued*)

Table 5.1 Characteristics of the studies included in the systematic review. (*Continued*)

Sl. no.	Study	Method	Conditions	Major findings
14	[33]	Mixed-methods retrospective observational study. N = 2194	Chronic Pain	Users with chronic pain showed significantly greater engagement with Wysa compared to those without chronic pain. Significant improvements in depression and anxiety symptoms after use. Users disengaged most often from the same tools they engaged with most (e.g., gratitude, sleep meditations, thought recording), suggesting potential limitations in maintaining long-term engagement. Helpful features: nonjudgmental space, Some users expressed a need for more direct human interaction, suggesting that AI-driven support alone may not be adequate for sustained emotional support.
15	[29]	Single-arm study, quantitative and qualitative analysis of feedback N = 30	Depressive symptoms	Useful Features: The mobile app was easy to use, accessible offline, and supported proactive skill building. Gamification, interactivity (enjoyable), and personalization enhanced engagement. High completion rates (80%) suggest strong adherence. Unhelpful: some users reported dizziness, dissociation, and difficulty integrating it into daily routines.

(*Continued*)

Table 5.1 Characteristics of the studies included in the systematic review. (*Continued*)

Sl. no.	Study	Method	Conditions	Major findings
16	[22]	System design and user perception (N = 37,169), controlled experiment (N = 1284)	Not a specific illness is addressed	Chatbots can simulate empathic support using peer-generated responses but are rated significantly lower than human responses. Users preferred responses from peers over the agent's responses, even when both were identical (framed the message as human-led or machine-generated). Helpful features: The use of real peer-generated responses made interactions feel more personal, and short-format interactions made the support scalable, filtering harmful content, and identifying users in crisis. Unhelpful features: Lacked perceived authenticity, lack of long-term interactions, short responses limited emotional depth.

(*Continued*)

Table 5.1 Characteristics of the studies included in the systematic review. (*Continued*)

Sl. no.	Study	Method	Conditions	Major findings
17	[39]	Observational, pre–post study design (12 wk) N = 778	Suicidal ideation	Significant reduction in suicidal ideation. Estimated 30.49% reduction in suicide attempts and deaths by suicide was observed based on previously established data linking Patient Health Questionnaire-9 SI scores to suicide outcomes. More frequent engagement with the therapy (more days per week) was associated with greater reductions in SI. Older age was linked to lower SI levels, and individuals with recurrent major depressive episodes had higher SI levels throughout treatment. Helpful features: Therapist support, evidence-based interventions (CBT, mindfulness, etc.), diverse therapy modules (mindfulness, negative cognition, mood regulation, emotion regulation, self-compassion, social functioning, sleep, and nutrition), daily exercises, psychoeducation videos, remote and scalable, anonymity, and emergency protocols for participants with worsening symptoms. Unhelpful features: limited peer interaction, excludes high-risk patients, and therapist time constraints.

(*Continued*)

Table 5.1 Characteristics of the studies included in the systematic review. (*Continued*)

Sl. no.	Study	Method	Conditions	Major findings
18	[30]	Single arm, open pilot study N = 12	Used as a blended therapy tool for the treatment of depression.	Rated high in usability, quality, and user satisfaction; all participants would use it again and recommend it. App exercises were integrated into therapy, but the extent of integration varied. Situational analysis was the most frequently used feature. Variation in module completion (1–7 per participants), lower engagement with longer exercises, and limited therapist guidance. Helpful features: Multiple-choice format reduced typing effort, situational analysis was well-integrated into therapy, self-management, and autonomy. Unhelpful features: Long duration exercises, modules were inconsistently integrated into therapy. There was no in-app saving option for entries (users had to take screenshots), and no therapist training on blended use.

(*Continued*)

Table 5.1 Characteristics of the studies included in the systematic review. (*Continued*)

Sl. no.	Study	Method	Conditions	Major findings
19	[36]	Qualitative exploratory study N = 10 (age group 12–18 y)	For adolescents recovering from concussion	Adolescents developed therapeutic alliances and social presence. Two key features: Guides' backgrounds (knowledge of concussions, psychology, and mindfulness) and guides' voices (calm, soothing tone increased connection). Helpful features: Audio narration by real mindfulness guides: increased connection and engagement, and SMS support from a coach Unhelpful features: Participants suggested adding photos of guides to increase social presence; they wanted more personalized feedback from the guides, and some participants found it hard to stay engaged without real-time human interaction.
20	[23]	Pilot clinical trial, 8-wk duration intervention N = 49	Chronic pain	Median retention of 51 d, significantly higher than the 4–16 d seen in other digital health interventions. Users who engaged with morning check-ins showed longer retention Users formed a therapeutic alliance with the CA, comparable to in-person psychotherapy. Helpful features: Personalization, behavioral activation, structured check-ins, and weekly engagement reports and roadmap for guidance. Lack of motivation for self-guided interventions.

(*Continued*)

Table 5.1 Characteristics of the studies included in the systematic review. (*Continued*)

Sl. no.	Study	Method	Conditions	Major findings
21	[37]	Qualitative analysis N = 184	Postpartum depression	Coaching support was highly valued (real-person coaching through telephone) Participants found elements such as videos, self-reflection exercises, and self-care strategies beneficial. Helpful features: Program accessibility, content, and supportive interactions with the coach. Unhelpful features: Limited coaching sessions, some participants found it hard to pinpoint whether improvements came from the app's structured content or the coaching calls.
22	[24]	Randomized controlled trial (10 wk) N = 166	Psychological distress	No significant difference in psychological distress between the intervention and control groups, the intervention did not improve working alliance or real relationship levels The intervention group showed a decrease in the genuineness dimension of the real relationship. High dropout rate in the intervention group, with those who dropped out reporting lower real relationship quality and less emotional disclosure. Helpful features: Self-assessment tools promoted reflection on emotional reactions and helped to raise awareness of emotional responses.

(*Continued*)

Table 5.1 Characteristics of the studies included in the systematic review. (*Continued*)

Sl. no.	Study	Method	Conditions	Major findings
23	[25]	Unblinded randomized controlled trial N = 192	Postpartum mental health (study did not focus on clinical population)	The chatbot group showed a greater decrease in depression symptoms compared to usual care. No significant differences were found between groups on anxiety or Edinburgh Postnatal Depression Scale. 91% of chatbot users were satisfied or highly satisfied with the tool. 80% of participants were comfortable with using a mobile app for mood management. Helpful features: Evidence-based interventions (CBT and IPT), accessible and cost-effective, mood-tracking functionality allows users to identify patterns, and crisis detection (this is Woebot feature, not a part of the intervention in this study). Lack of direct human support was reported as unhelpful.

(*Continued*)

Table 5.1 Characteristics of the studies included in the systematic review. (*Continued*)

Sl. no.	Study	Method	Conditions	Major findings
24	[26]	Randomized controlled trial N = 231	Symptoms of depression, anxiety, and stress	Alert-based features (motivational messages and symptom-tracking reminders) were the most commonly used. Use of these features was associated with significant improvements in anxiety and functional impairment. Reminders received *via* SMS were more strongly associated with symptom improvement than email reminders, though the difference was not statistically significant. Participants showed higher engagement with the app compared to other eMental health interventions. Module completion rates were low likely due to the lack of mobile access for modules and the rigid "tunneled" progression. Helpful features: SMS alerts and symptom tracking. Unhelpful features: Limited module access through mobile (only web-based access) and tunneled module progression

Appendix 2

Table 5.2 Characteristics of mobile apps mentioned in the reviewed studies.

Sl. no.	Apps	Used for (from user feedback)	Functions	Study
1	Headspace	To better manage mood and to feel calmer To help with sleep and anaxiety To support overcoming challenges with anxiety To reduce daily anxiety and stress symptoms by calming self General support for well-being To reduce anxiety	Meditation	[34]
2	Brain in hand	To ground self when dissociating To support overcoming challenges with anxiety	Traffic light system to manage mental health and access support	[34]
3	Insight Timer	To help relax before bed	Meditation	[34]
4	Calm	To feel calmer To improve focus and sleep To improve sleep	Meditation and sleep	[34]
5	Balance	To reduce daily anxiety and stress symptoms by calming self	Meditation	[34]
6	My Life	To reduce daily anxiety and stress symptoms by calming self	Meditation	[34]

(Continued)

Table 5.2 Characteristics of mobile apps mentioned in the reviewed studies. (*Continued*)

Sl. no.	Apps	Used for (from user feedback)	Functions	Study
7	Pixel	Document thoughts to identify patterns and mood fluctuations To help with anxiety by getting thoughts down and to relax	Journaling and mood tracking	[34]
8	Habit tracking	To keep on track of positive activities	Behavior tracking	[34]
9	Clear fear		Anxiety management	[34]
10	Calm harm	To reduce self-harm	Manage urges to self-harm	[34]
11	Cove		Music therapy	[34]
12	I am sober		Habit tracking and motivation	[34]
13	Wysa	To track mood fluctuations and patterns To manage anxiety symptoms For pain management (chronic pain) To support those who had sleep difficulties	Chatbot	[23, 31, 33–35]
14	Tomo		Mindfulness	[34]
15	Today I am	To help build an emotional language to name feelings	Increase emotional literacy	[34]
16	Smiling mind	To stay calm and be able to clear mind and distract self when feeling low or anxious	Meditation	[34]

(*Continued*)

Table 5.2 Characteristics of mobile apps mentioned in the reviewed studies. (*Continued*)

Sl. no.	Apps	Used for (from user feedback)	Functions	Study
17	Abide	To stay calm and be able to clear mind and distract self when feeling low or anxious	Meditation	[34]
18	Health Assured		Track health	[34]
19	Self-help for anxiety management	To develop strategies to apply when alone	Anxiety management skills	[34]
20	For me	To develop strategies to apply when alone	Self-help information	[34]
21	MOST+ (Enhanced Moderated Online Social Therapy)	To provide web-based counseling, interactive therapy, and peer support	Web-based interventions, online peer support groups, and web-based counseling	[27]
22	Insight App	To develop skills to manage stress and regulate emotions	cognitive behavioral therapy (CBT), acceptance and commitment therapy, and mindfulness-based interventions	[17]
23	Life Flex	To increase psychological flexibility and positive affect on anxiety and depression in adults	Self-help techniques and therapist assistance through video chat	[18]
24	Woebot	Conversational agent	CBT techniques provided through text-based messages, provides psychoeducational content and mood-tracking features	[25, 28, 38]

(*Continued*)

Table 5.2 Characteristics of mobile apps mentioned in the reviewed studies. (*Continued*)

Sl. no.	Apps	Used for (from user feedback)	Functions	Study
25	MYLO	Relational agents support psychological well-being by facilitating reflective conversations	Method of Levels (MOL) therapy uses curious questioning to help users explore their thoughts, gain new insights, and develop their own understanding of their problems	[12]
26	XiaoE	To provide automated mental health support *via* chatbot interaction	Screening, self-help, and CBT-based support	[19]
27	ERICA	To teach cognitive emotion regulation strategies	Conversational agents that provide interactive dialogues and psychoeducation	[20]
28	Fido	To reduce subclinical depressive and anxiety symptoms	Chatbot that uses CBT techniques such as Socratic questioning, cognitive distortion identification, and general psychoeducation	[21]

(*Continued*)

Table 5.2 Characteristics of mobile apps mentioned in the reviewed studies. (*Continued*)

Sl. no.	Apps	Used for (from user feedback)	Functions	Study
29	Spark	To reduce depressive symptoms in adolescents	Self-guided digital intervention combining a mobile app and virtual reality experiences. CBT-based content. Interactive, gamified, and personalized modules focused on skill building, symptom management, and emotion regulation	[29]
30	Koko	To promote emotional resilience by facilitating cognitive reappraisal and supportive interactions	Chatbot (KokoBot) that guides users through cognitive restructuring techniques and moderates peer exchanges	[22]
31	CBASPath	To use between therapy sessions and in-session discussions, as a blended therapy tool For patients undergoing CBASP for persistent depressive disorder	A digital augmentation of CBASP therapy, psychoeducation, transference hypothesis, interpersonal exercises, etc., and situational analysis exercises	[30]
32	4-wk mindfulness-based intervention	To equip patients with pain acceptance, stress management, and to help with concussion symptoms	A self-guided smartphone app that provides psychoeducation and mindfulness exercises narrated by trained mindfulness guides	[36]

(*Continued*)

Table 5.2 Characteristics of mobile apps mentioned in the reviewed studies. (*Continued*)

Sl. no.	Apps	Used for (from user feedback)	Functions	Study
33	MomMoodBooster	To help veteran women with postpartum depression	Structured content, internet-delivered CBT program and coaching calls	[37]
34	Internet-Based Routine Process Monitoring and Feedback System	To enhance self-monitoring of emotional reactions in individual psychotherapy sessions	A platform for self-assessment and promotes patient awareness of their emotional experiences during therapy	[24]
35	SimSimi	For general conversation	Open-domain social chatbot, not therapy-focused	[32]
36	Meru Health Program (MHP)	To reduce suicidal ideation, depression, and anxiety symptoms	Therapist-supported digital mental health intervention. Includes therapist-supported care, self-guided modules, daily exercises and emergency protocol	[39]
37	myCompass	To provides digital mental health intervention for mild to moderate depression, anxiety, and stress symptoms	Web and mobile based self-help intervention includes interactive psychotherapy modules, symptom tracking, motivational messages, and diary features	[26]

6

Future Directions: Toward a Digital Mental Health Ecosystem

Vinoth Kumar S.[1], Anand Bharathi S.[2*], S. Rajamohan[3] and D. Unika[1]

[1]PG and Research Department of Commerce, Patrician College of Arts and Science, Chennai, India
[2]Department of Management Studies, Jain University, Bangalore, India
[3]Department of Management Studies, Fatima College, Madurai, India

Abstract

The rapidly evolving field of digital mental health research is examined in this study, mainly due to technological advancements and the global consequences of COVID-19. It uses bibliometrics and a systematic literature review to understand the trends and determine future research opportunities. The flow diagram following the PRISMA methodology shows results for literature selection, which exposes a drastically increasing research output after 2020, although older works still dominate the citation crown. The field is shaped by several journals, such as *JMIR Mental Health* and the *Journal of Consulting and Clinical Psychology* (*JOCACP*), whereas the *Games for Health Journal* (*GFHJ*) brings newly emerging intersections with the digital gaming world. The most researched areas of interest include depression, anxiety, mHealth, telehealth, artificial intelligence (AI) interventions, and, more recently, digital phenotyping and AI ethics. The study also notes a globally expanding field with significant contributions from the United States, New Zealand, Kenya, and Australia. An evaluation of 1185 studies from SCOPUS and Web of Science showcases a cohesive, innovative research community. The study underlines the growing need for collaboration between fields and further exploration of these aspects of other health systems to ensure the effective integration of digital tools as interventions in mental health across healthcare systems.

***Keywords*:** Digital mental health, mental health ecosystem, bibliometric analysis, thematic analysis, systematic literature review

**Corresponding author*: nndbhrthi@gmail.com

Raghavendra M. Devadas, Vani Hiremani, Preethi, Praveen Gujjar, Sapna R. and Manoj Shettar (eds.) Psychiatry and Technology, (161–194) © 2026 Scrivener Publishing LLC

6.1 Introduction

The use of technologies such as apps, wearables, artificial intelligence (AI), and telehealth platforms to assist in assessing, diagnosing, treating, and preventing illnesses is referred to as digital mental health [1–3]. With the continuing increase of mental health disorders worldwide, digital solutions as possible interventions may provide better access and be more cost-effective and scalable [4–6]. Such technologies address shortcomings of conventional mental healthcare by overcoming geographic restrictions, stigma, and shortage of providers.

In the modern era, the numbers associated with mental illnesses such as depression, anxiety, and posttraumatic stress disorder have been rising at an alarming rate globally [7–10]. Although fundamental, the traditionally known systems and units of healthcare struggle to keep up with the ever-increasing demand for mental healthcare services [11]. Due to factors such as high expense, scarce providers, increasing cost of treatment, and long wait times, many people are unable to receive necessary care promptly [12–15]. An individual can now receive the required support irrespective of their geographical location. This approach addresses the aforementioned barriers more innovatively using technologies based on the internet [16].

The current healthcare system highlights that digital mental health helps facilitate access to care, enable earlier interventions, and tailor treatments [3, 6, 17]. With progress in machine learning, data analytics, and telehealth technologies, digital platforms can offer real-time monitoring, evidence-based practices, and predictive analytics of mental health as foreseen [18–20]. Enhancing accessibility and the quality of mental healthcare services, these tools have made remarkable strides. Applications such as Headspace and Calm provide guided mindfulness meditations and stress reduction exercises [21], and AI-driven platforms have started providing therapeutic conversations, such as Woebot, which bases its chats on cognitive behavioral therapy (CBT) [22, 23]. BetterHelp and Talkspace offer telehealth services where users are connected to licensed therapists and have their therapy sessions *via* video calls, giving people who otherwise might not have had the opportunity greater access to therapy [24, 25].

The growth of digital mental health dates back to self-help resources but now includes teletherapy, AI interventions, and advanced mental health monitoring systems [26, 27]. These technologies were further propelled into use due to the COVID-19 pandemic as they showcased their ability to provide care when in-person visits were not a possibility [28–30]. Now, machine learning algorithms are personalizing treatment plans, and wearables track physiological data in real time to ascertain mental well-being [31].

The scope of digital mental health encompasses concerns to further regions as individuals can access services, seek help, and receive better response times, all from the privacy of their homes, eliminating the fear of being stigmatized and making help more accessible. Healthcare digital platforms assist with diagnosis, treatment, and pharmacological and nonpharmacological monitoring, boosting patient care. Lastly, digital mental health solutions answer the long-standing issue of offering affordable services for scaling the response to the global mental health crisis, providing options to the policymakers of the sector.

Even considering the prospects it holds, digital mental health is stunted due to a lack of data privacy, underregulation, and insufficient digital literacy. Regardless, any emerging technologies in this field need to be effective and equitable, accessible to everyone, and, above all, implemented ethically, necessitating considering the relevant social factors.

6.1.1 Chapter's Aim

This chapter aims to study the digital mental health research domain and establish its future trajectory. The chapter will analyze the advancement and proliferation of digital mental health research using bibliometric analysis and systematic literature review (SLR). From publication and citation practices to author and institutional collaborations, the chapter will report major milestones alongside pivotal contributors within the field. It will examine the evolution of thematic research areas and the turning points, using tools such as the thematic map and thematic evolution to display these shifts. In addition, the chapter will examine the impact of the most cited sources on digital mental health technologies and elucidate prevalent research themes through the word cloud and co-occurrence network. Finally, the chapter will outline evolving research themes and recommend actionable steps to sustain and deepen the interest in the field. The findings will be presented alongside the PRISMA flowchart, yearly publications alongside annual citations, and collaboration network, as well as the figures, charts, and tables, which will depict the comprehensive landscape of the field's evolution and prospective avenues of research.

6.1.2 Overview of the Methodology

The PRISMA flowchart (Figure 6.1) presented by Moher *et al.* [32] exemplifies the integrative approach using bibliometric analysis as described by Donthu *et al.* [33] and Ellegaard and Wallin [34], and an SLR conducted by Pati and Lorusso [35], as well as Sauer and Seuring [36] helps to highlight the significant contributions in digital mental health research. The current study obtained data from SCOPUS and Web of Science, which are recognized as primary scholarly databases [37, 38]. The first search containing "digital mental health" produced 2439 records. After applying filters based on document type (articles and reviews), the number was narrowed down to 2044, which was subsequently refined to 2033 after incorporating English-only studies.

One of the crucial steps concerning methodology was performing data analysis using R, where both databases were combined into one dataset. Data cleaning procedures removing identical entries were initially conducted in R, streamlining 848 duplicate rows of data that hindered information quality. Of these 1185 complete bibliographic datasets retained for bibliometric and systematic literature analysis, only the meticulously compiled dataset was curated. Digitally poring over assembled documents proves valid the precision evaluating

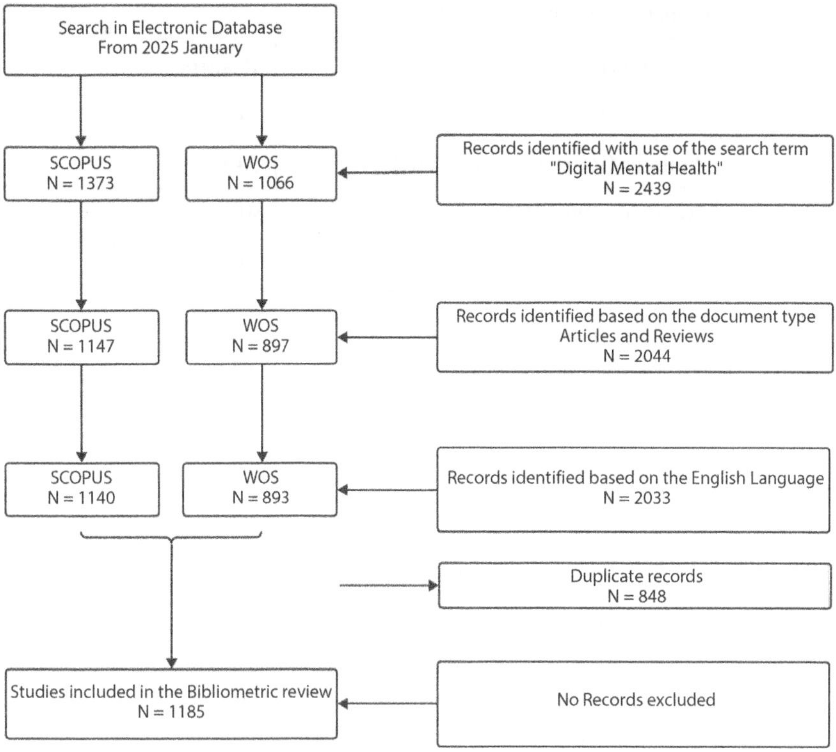

Figure 6.1 PRISMA flowchart. **Source:** Developed by the authors using PRISMA framework.

trends, the body of work, and the direction of work undertaken to analyze the holistic mental health digital interventions system.

6.2 Research Trends and Key Metrics

6.2.1 Summary Statistics

The bibliometric analysis of 1185 documents published between 2013 and 2025 provides a comprehensive overview of research trends (Table 6.1) in digital mental health. The study draws insights from 349 sources, including journals, books, and conference proceedings, demonstrating diverse scholarly contributions. The keyword analysis reveals 914 Keywords Plus (ID) and 812 Author's Keywords (DE),

Table 6.1 Summary statistics.

Description	Results
Documents	1185
Sources (journals, books, etc.)	349
Keywords Plus (ID)	914
Author's keywords (DE)	812
Period	2013:2025
Average citations per document	2.778
Authors	5069
Authors of single-authored documents	34
Authors of multiauthored documents	5035
Single-authored documents	36
Documents per author	0.2337
Authors per document	4.2776
Coauthors per document	6.48

Source: Developed by the authors based on R.

indicating a rich and evolving terminological landscape within this field. The research domain exhibits a moderate citation impact, with an average of 2.778 citations per document, reflecting the growing academic interest and influence of digital mental health studies.

The collaboration trends indicate that the networked research community is well-connected. The body of knowledge has been contributed to by 5069 authors, of which only 34 published documents that were not coauthored, meaning 5035 authors participated in multiauthored research. This is corroborated by the low ratio of single-authorship documents and their high multiauthored counterparts, revealing a focus on collaborative research. Single-authored documents totaled 36 of 1185. That equates to roughly 3% single authorship, which signals overwhelming multiauthorship and collaboration. An author in the body of knowledge averages 0.2337 documents, but each document has around 4.2776 authors showing deep multidisciplinary interaction. The average coauthorship per document metric of 6.48 reinforces an interdisciplinary collaboration figure of digital mental health research that pulls from psychology, computer science, healthcare, and AI.

6.2.2 Annual Publications and Citations

As the annual publication trends (Table 6.2) suggest, the research output concerning the sector of digital mental health has been gaining unprecedented interest, hence the rise in publications over the last few years. The overall output of published articles went up continuously, reaching its highest point in 2024 with 371 articles and also publishing 261 and 207 in 2023 and 2022, respectively. This clearly shows the surge of focus around the concepts of digital mental health, primarily due to ever-evolving technology, the surge of

Table 6.2 Annual publications.

Year	No. of articles	Mean TC per article
2024	371	0.32
2023	261	0.84
2022	207	2.37
2021	170	3.04
2020	83	14.02
2019	41	13.05
2025	24	0.21
2017	13	8.38
2018	11	4.82
2016	3	27.00

Source: Developed by the authors based on R.

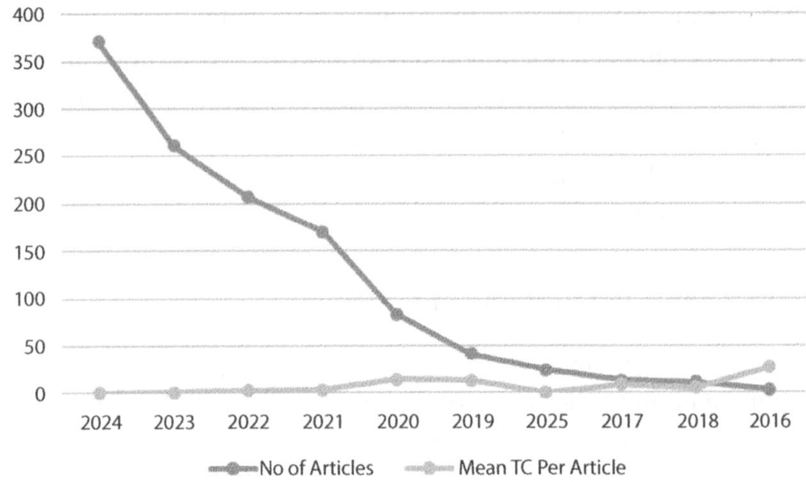

Figure 6.2 Top annual publications and citations. **Source:** Developed by the authors based on R.

global mental health issues, and the COVID-19 pandemic, among other things.

According to total citation (TC) metrics (Figure 6.2), however, the per-article averages follow a different path. Citation rates are higher for older publications (e.g., 2016: 27 citations per article, 2020: 14.02, 2019: 13.05), whereas more recent publications have lower citation counts (2024: 0.32, 2023: 0.84, 2025: 0.21). This illustrates a well-known pattern in bibliometrics where older articles have had more time to accrue citations. In contrast, newer works have yet to be fully recognized by the academic community. The sharp increase in publications starting in 2020 corresponds to the COVID-19 pandemic, which accelerated the integration of digital mental health tools. The additional output in 2021 (170 articles), 2022 (207 articles), and 2023 (261 articles) also demonstrates the growing scope of the field, although more recent studies tend to have a limited citation impact. As for the 2025 projection, the 24 articles and 0.21 citations per article are barebones and assume publication and citation growth following the report.

6.2.3 Top Cited Articles

Analyzing the most cited articles (Table 6.3) in the context of digital mental health research reveals vital Myrick's [39] work on digital mental health and COVID-19: Using Technology Today to Accelerate the Curve on Access and Quality Published in *JMIR Mental Health* is cited 569 times. It is remarkable how the COVID-19 expenditure triggers the research of digital mental health tools, showcasing the need for tech interventions. Subsequently, Schueller [40] investigated the application of digital mental health tools for marginalized and underserved populations, published in *Current Treatment Options in Psychiatry* (*CTOIP*), with 155 citations. This research highlights how utilizing digital means can transform mental health services for marginalized populations. In the same vein, Graham [41] and Torous [42] analyzed the implementation and the scale of evidence-based digital treatment to remotely accessible healthcare services and infrastructure, *American Psychologist* (*AP*), 108 and 83, respectively. These data point to the increasing attention paid to mental healthcare provision through digital means.

The *Internet Interventions* (*II*) article by Lattie [43] published a study on Intellicare, a mental health app suite, and was cited 81 times. His citation count, much greater than that of his peers who published around the same time, demonstrates ongoing interest in mobile app–based interventions despite them being published much earlier. Likewise, Pine [44] performed a systematic review of the use of casual video games and their relationship with anxiety, depression, and stress in the *GFHJ*, receiving 75 citations. Moreover, Osborn [45] assessed single-session digital interventions for adolescent mental health in Kenya, published in the *JOCACP*, accumulating 74 citations. This highlights the potential of digital interventions globally, especially in regions with fewer resources. Parker [46] analyzed the use of mental health applications and the implications of privacy issues in the *International Journal of Law and Psychiatry* (*IJOLAP*) and was cited 73 times. This suggests that the debate on data protection in mental healthcare systems is becoming more prevalent.

Table 6.3 Top cited articles.

Author	Year	Title	Source	TC
Myrick	2020	"Digital Mental Health and COVID-19: Using Technology Today to Accelerate the Curve on Access and Quality Tomorrow"	*JMIR Mental Health*	569
Schueller	2019	"Use of Digital Mental Health for Marginalized and Underserved Populations"	*Current Treatment Options in Psychiatry*	155
Graham	2020	"Implementation Strategies for Digital Mental Health Interventions in Health Care Settings"	*American Psychologist*	108
Torous	2020	"Scaling Evidence-Based Treatments Through Digital Mental Health"	*American Psychologist*	83
Lattie	2016	"Uptake and Usage of Intellicare: A Publicly Available Suite of Mental Health and Well-being Apps"	*Internet Interventions*	81
Pine	2020	"The Effects of Casual Videogames on Anxiety, Depression, Stress, and Low Mood: A Systematic Review"	*Games for Health Journal*	75
Osborn	2020	"Single-Session Digital Intervention for Adolescent Depression, Anxiety, and Well-being: Outcomes of a Randomized Controlled Trial With Kenyan Adolescents"	*Journal of Consulting and Clinical Psychology*	74

(*Continued*)

Table 6.3 Top cited articles. (*Continued*)

Author	Year	Title	Source	TC
Parker	2019	"How Private Is Your Mental Health App Data? An Empirical Study of Mental Health App Privacy Policies and Practices"	*International Journal of Law and Psychiatry*	73
Balcombe	2021	"Digital Mental Health Challenges and The Horizon Ahead for Solutions"	*JMIR Mental Health*	62
Wasil	2020	"Reassessing Evidence-Based Content in Popular Smartphone Apps for Depression and Anxiety: Developing and Applying User-Adjusted Analyses"	*Journal of Consulting and Clinical Psychology*	56

Source: Developed by the authors.

Moreover, Balcombe [1] incorporated the hurdles and prospective advancements of digital mental health in its scope, which has been cited 62 times, highlighting the lack of sustainable and practical solutions. Lastly, Wasil [47] analyzed the evidence-based approaches to content in mental health smartphone applications and was cited 56 times, stressing the need for validated scientific interventions within the *JOCACP*. The citations signify emerging research concerns such as unrestricted access to care among underserved groups, the COVID-19–influenced digital care delivery model, the use of mobile applications, the trust and safety framework, and the future of mental healthcare and technology integration. These research activities inform the evolution of digital mental health and are important for decision-makers, care providers, and technology innovators.

6.2.4 Three-Field Paths

The three-field path analysis (Figure 6.3) showcases the complex patterns of interaction between authors (AU), keywords (DE), and sources (SO) in digital mental health research. Significant contributors identified are Torous J, Gleeson J, Forman-Hoffman V, Alvarez-Jimenez M, Schueller S, Mohr D, and Bucci S, prominently Torous J, demonstrating profound engagement with the research. The authors' interconnectedness suggests synergistic collaboration in digital mental health research. Primary axes of focus include "digital mental health," "mental health," "depression," "anxiety," "mHealth," "COVID-19," "telehealth," "technology," and "artificial intelligence." The use of "COVID-19" as a keyword reasserts the pandemic's influence on accelerating research in digital mental health interventions.

Furthermore, the use of terminology such as "digital mental health interventions," "telemedicine," and "adolescents" illustrates the expanding focus on specific interventions and targeted populations. Most of the research is published within the journalistic domain of the *Journal of Technology in Behavioral Science*, *JMIR Formative Research*, *Frontiers in Psychology* (*FIP*), *JMIR Mental Health*, *Behavior Research and Therapy* (*BRAT*), *JOCACP*, and *Journal of Medical Internet Research* (*JMIR*). The *JMIR* journals seem to be leading in this area, which mirrors the growth of interest in online and internet health research. It is fueled by technology-centric mental healthcare

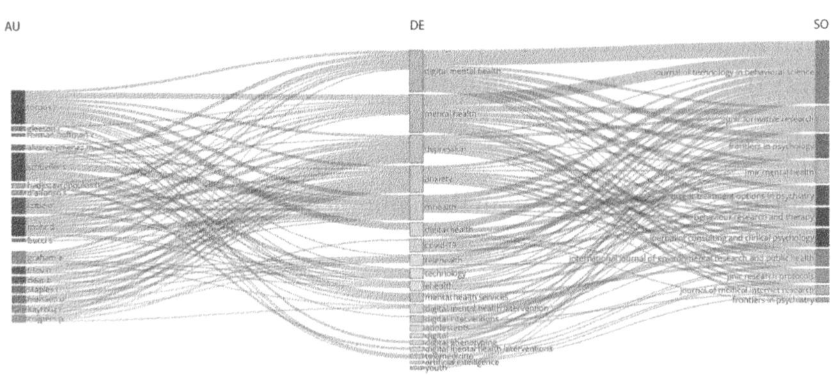

Figure 6.3 Three-field paths. **Source:** Developed by the authors based on R.

services with important authorship and intensive publishing activity in specialized behavioral science and medical internet research journals. These results also emphasize the further increase in the importance of remote care solutions as exacerbated by global health crises, such as the COVID-19 pandemic.

6.3 Influential Contributors and Research Impact

6.3.1 Most Cited Sources with Indexes and Top Cited Sources

The citation analysis (Table 6.4) of the leading contributors in the domain of research related to digital mental health indicates that *JMIR Mental Health* is the most cited journal, having 749 TCs, 106 published papers (NP) with an *H* index of 7 and a *G* index of 27. This demonstrates that *JMIR Mental Health* exerts the most significant influence and has the widest coverage in the field, showing that it has a foundational role in publishing research on digital mental health interventions. Subsequent to *JMIR Mental Health*, *CTOIP* and the *JOCACP* have also emerged as major contributors, having 319 and 244 TCs, respectively, and *H* index of 6. Their moderate impact indicates that these psychiatry and clinical psychology journals are expanding their readership to include digital mental health research. Other sources of interest include *AP*, *FIP*, *GFHJ*, and *IJOLAP*. Of these, *FIP* possesses considerable prominence, having published 13 papers with an *H* index of 8, suggesting ongoing scholarly activity in digital mental health.

The emergence of the *GFHJ* also underlines the increasing importance of digital gaming as an intervention for mental health issues (Figure 6.4). Other journals, including *BRAT*, *II*, and *Cognitive and Behavioral Practice* (*CABP*), have lower citation metrics but still make valuable contributions. These journals are known as *II*, *CABP*, and BRAT, and they collectively possess lower citation influence (*II*'s TC = 81, *H* index = 1), a metric that displays steadily increasing impact. *II* is at the very bottom with the least claim to influence. The analysis of *JMIR Mental Health* dominates other regional mental

Table 6.4 Most cited sources and their indexes.

Source	TC	NP	H index	G index
JMIR Mental Health	749	106	7	27
CTOIP	319	9	6	9
JOCACP	244	8	6	8
AP	200	4	4	4
FIP	141	13	8	11
GFHJ	124	3	2	3
IJOLAP	115	2	2	2
BRAT	108	7	5	7
CABP	100	7	5	7
II	81	1	1	1

Source: Developed by the authors based on R.

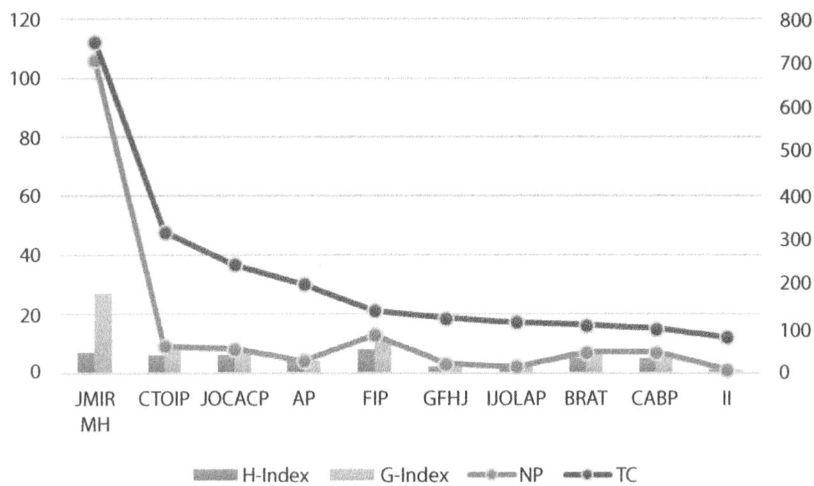

Figure 6.4 Top cited sources: Publications and indexes. **Source:** Developed by the authors based on R. *JMIR MH, JMIR Mental Health; CTOIP, Current Treatment Options in Psychiatry; JOCACP, Journal of Consulting and Clinical Psychology; AP, American Psychologist; FIP, Frontiers in Psychology; GFHJ, Games for Health Journal; IJOLAP, International Journal of Law and Psychiatry; BRAT, Behaviour Research and Therapy; CABP, Cognitive and Behavioral Practice; II, Internet Interventions.*

health journals, along with older psychiatry and psychology journals. The inclusion of behavioral, cognitive, and digitally oriented health therapy journals indicates a blend of modern approaches into deep-rooted frameworks of mental healthcare. The difference in citation values also displays variation in publishing avenues from general psychology and psychiatry to more focused digital and intervention journals.

6.3.2 Leading Authors, Affiliations, and Countries

The examination of the leading authors, their affiliations, and countries regarding their citation influence sheds light on the critical contributors to digital mental health (Table 6.5, Figures 6.5 and 6.6). Myrick, from Los Angeles County in the United States, emerges as the leading figure with a whopping 569 TCs across three publications

Table 6.5 Leading authors, affiliations, and countries: Categorized by citation influence.

Authors	Affiliations	Countries	TC	NP
Myrick	Los Angeles County	USA	569	3
Schueller	School of Social and Behavioral Sciences Gateway Irvine	USA	155	32
Graham	Northwestern University	USA	108	14
Torous	Harvard Medical School	USA	83	40
Lattie	Northwestern University	USA	81	23
Pine	Victoria University of Wellington	New Zealand	75	5
Osborn	Harvard University and Shamiri Institute	Kenya	74	1
Parker	University of Sydney	Australia	73	1
Balcombe	Griffith University	Australia	62	8
Wasil	University of Pennsylvania	USA	56	9

Source: Developed by the authors based on R.

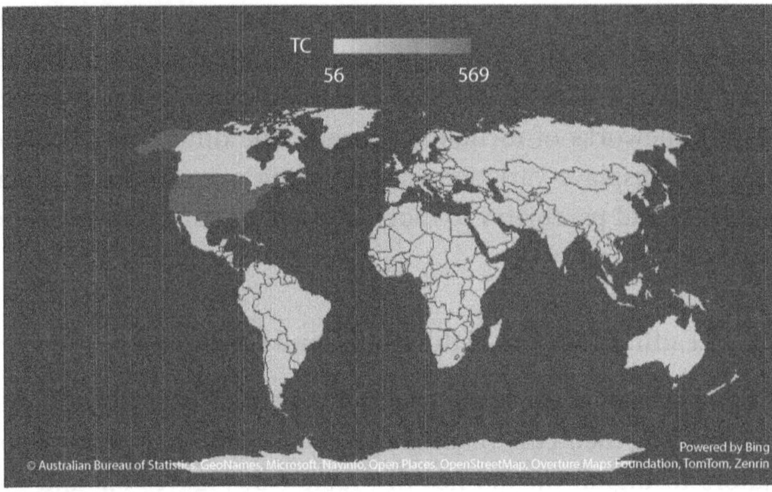

Figure 6.5 Authors' countries with top citation records and publications. **Source:** Developed by the authors based on R.

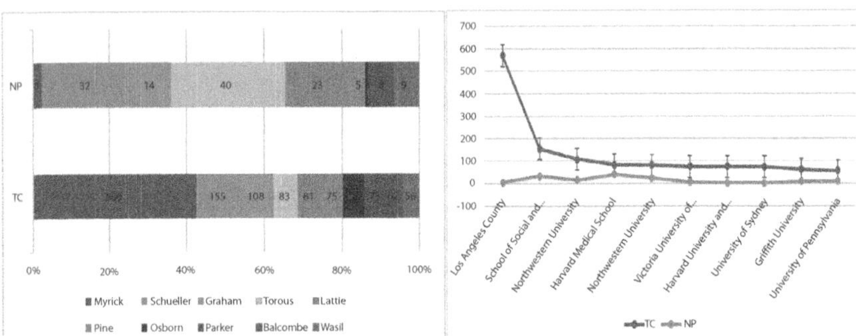

Figure 6.6 Authors and authors' affiliations with top citation records and publications. **Source:** Developed by the authors based on R.

(NP = 3), which is a remarkable impact per publication. This indicates that Myrick's work has been extensively cited, which might not be surprising considering the limited number of publications. Among the most prolific Torous (Harvard Medical School, USA) and Schueller (School of Social and Behavioral Sciences Gateway Irvine, USA), who claim 40 and 32 publications, relatively low TC counts (83, 155, respectively) indicate a relatively poor impact per paper ratio. Moreover, Graham (Northwestern University, USA) and Lattie (Northwestern University, USA) significantly contribute and demonstrate the presence of Northwestern University in this research field.

On an international scale, the digital mental health research landscape has been influenced by Pine (Victoria University of Wellington, New Zealand), Osborn (Harvard University and Shamiri Institute, Kenya), Parker (University of Sydney, Australia), and Balcombe (Griffith University, Australia). The high citation count (74) by Osborn from a single publication points toward some groundbreaking or at least highly relevant research. Parker (University of Sydney, Australia) follows a similar pattern with 73 citations from just one paper, indicating some highly impactful studies. The United States dominates the digital mental health research field. Six of the 10 authors with the most significant influence are from American institutions.

Nevertheless, the presence of New Zealand, Kenyan, and Australian researchers highlights growing international participation in these studies. The gap in the impact of publication and citation between these authors indicates a vast difference in scholarly approaches, with some striving to maximize output. In contrast, others achieve fame through fewer highly cited studies. As is always the case, an evolving field such as digital mental health will have fierce publishing coupled with highly impactful individual contributions, or vice versa.

6.4 Thematic Insights and Concept Evolution

6.4.1 Most Frequent Words and Word Cloud

The keyword analysis sheds light on the main themes and developments in the research area of digital mental health (Table 6.6 and Figure 6.7). Notably, "digital mental health" is the most cited phrase in the analysis, which occurred 87 times. This powerfully illustrates that the primary concern of the field is to use technology to promote mental health. This is almost the same with "mental health," which

Table 6.6 Most frequent words.

Words	Occurrences
Digital mental health	87
Mental health	80
Depression	32
Anxiety	29
mHealth	29
COVID-19	23
Digital health	20
Digital mental health interventions	16
Telehealth	15
eHealth	11

Source: Developed by the authors based on R.

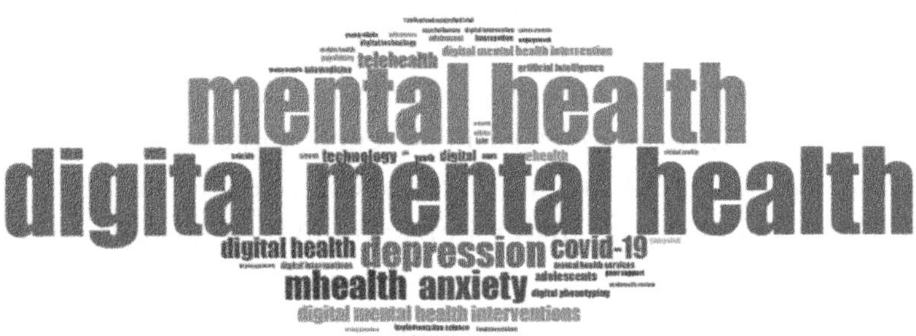

Figure 6.7 Word cloud. **Source:** Developed by the authors based on R.

has 80 occurrences, meaning that mental health issues remain the primary focus within the research ecosystem. Important mental health conditions also include "depression" with 32 occurrences and "anxiety" with 29 occurrences. This suggests a strong focus on researching to help treat these common psychological disorders through digital technology. The presence of "mHealth" (29 occurrences), "eHealth" (11 occurrences), and "digital health" (20 occurrences) shows that there is considerable attention given to mobile and electronic health technologies, further showing the focus on technological solutions to health problems.

The effects of the COVID-19 global pandemic on digital mental health are specific and noticeable, as "COVID-19" is cited an aggregate of 23 times. This shows how the pandemic fast-tracked the implementation of remote digital mental health services, especially regarding remote patient care and telehealth. Closely related words include "telehealth," cited 15 times, and "telemedicine," cited 7 times, emphasizing the growing dependence on online healthcare services.

The use of data-focused and AI-driven techniques for the assessment and treatment of mental health issues is being researched extensively, as seen by the specific terms "digital mental health interventions" (16 occurrences), "digital interventions" (7 occurrences), and "digital phenotyping" (8 occurrences). The mention of "artificial intelligence" (8 occurrences) indicates a growing adoption of AI in digital mental health studies and applications. Moreover, "adolescents" (10 occurrences) denotes an area of emerging interest within mental health dealing with younger people, indicating that digital interventions are designed for younger people because of their high-tech usage. "Mental health services" (7 occurrences) further endorse the use of digital means in expanding the availability of psychological services. The focus on depression and anxiety and the recent advancements in AI, telehealth, and digital techniques indicate that the sector is shifting toward more personalized care that is easier to access and relies on data.

6.4.2 Co-Occurrence Network

The co-occurrence network analysis (Figure 6.8) demonstrates important features and connections within the digital mental health research framework. The most important node, "digital mental health," captures its significance in the field. Connected concepts such as "apps," "implementation science," "virtual reality," and "digital psychiatry" showcase the focus on the use of technology in mental health interventions. A notable cluster includes mental health services, telehealth, and suicide prevention, which illustrates the

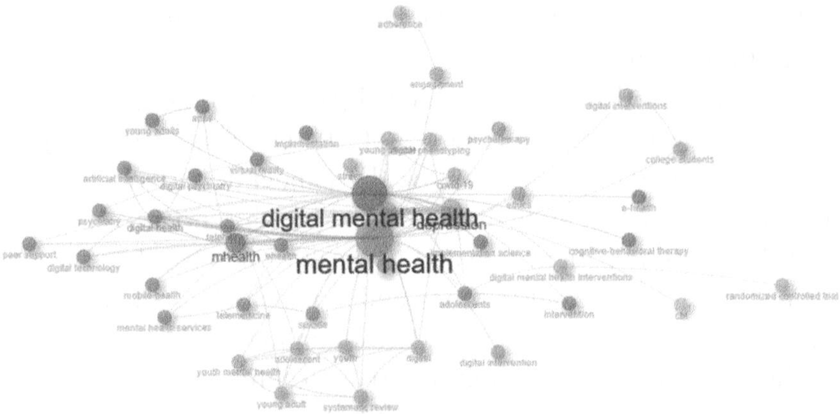

Figure 6.8 Co-occurrence network. **Source:** Developed by the authors based on R.

growing dependence on technological resources to enhance mental healthcare services. The mention of "telemedicine" and "mental health services" denotes the increasing adoption of remote healthcare services, a phenomenon that has surged due to the COVID-19 pandemic.

Another significant area of focus is mental illnesses such as depression and anxiety, which often overlap with "mHealth," "digital interventions," and "stress." This implies that some research is directed at creating and assessing digital solutions for treating these illnesses. The inclusion of "adolescents," "youth," and "young adults" within the network indicates a responsive interest in expanding mental healthcare services to younger age groups, considering their increased use of technology. Moreover, "digital health," "telehealth," "eHealth," and "artificial intelligence" create a distinct cluster, illustrating the advancing role of technology in mental health research. The emergence of "digital phenotyping" further suggests an inclination toward the use of data in the evaluation and treatment of mental health issues. The network also mentions "engagement," "adherence," and "randomized controlled trials," which serve as paradigms for evaluating the impact and effectiveness of the provided digital services. The inclusion of CBT portrays the increasing use of digital platforms to provide evidence-based mental healthcare services.

As expected, the co-occurrence network indicates the interdisciplinary approaches associated with digital mental health research, including technology, clinical psychology, and public health. Focused concerns of the findings highlight accessibility, effectiveness, and technological integration, which reveal digital mental health as an innovative frontier in modern mental healthcare.

6.4.3 Thematic Map and Evolution

The thematic map (Figure 6.9) offers an organized breakdown of areas of investigation under digital mental health by identifying niche themes, motor themes, essential themes, and emerging themes relative to their centrality and impact.

Basic themes (fundamental concepts in digital mental health)
The cluster of keywords forming "digital mental health" encompasses mental health, depression, anxiety, mHealth, and COVID-19, marking the foundational constituent of research in this area. Themes are fundamental to scholarly discourse and exhibit high

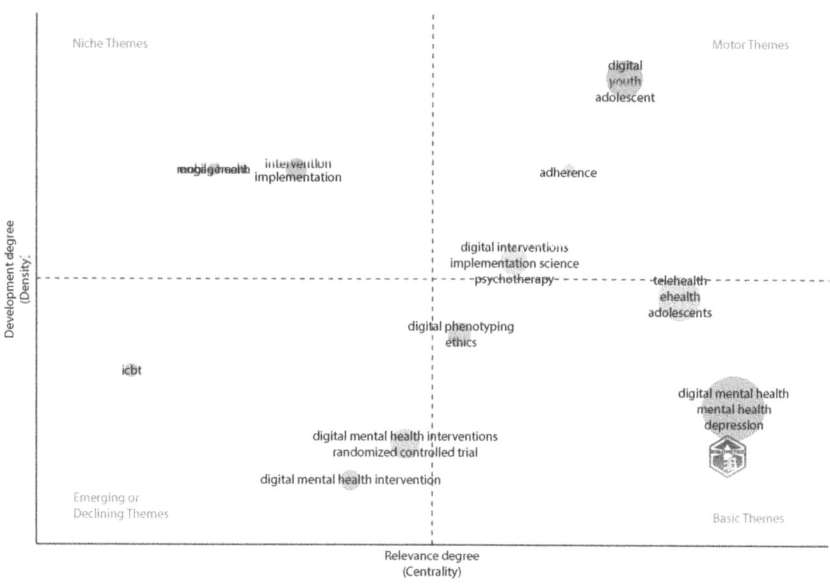

Figure 6.9 Thematic map. **Source:** Developed by the authors based on R.

betweenness centrality and PageRank. Focus on the COVID-19 pandemic underscores the heightened adoption of digital mental health tools during the crisis. The inclusion of "digital technology," "artificial intelligence," and "apps" within this cluster indicates that further advancements in technology will continue to transform the landscape of mental healthcare.

Motor themes (driving forces in digital mental health research)
These prominent and thoroughly developed topics motivate and propel other research areas in digital mental health. "Digital mental health interventions" and "telehealth" are essential motor themes, suggesting a high level of integration with healthcare systems. The existence of "eHealth," "telemedicine," "psychiatry," and "suicide" in this category indicates the utilization of mental health services, crisis intervention, and psychiatric services through digital means. Additionally, the "engagement" cluster stresses the crucial role of adherence and user participation toward achieving positive outcomes in these interventions.

Niche themes (specialized and emerging research areas)
Niche themes are less integrated into the core of digital mental health research but are important to analyze because of their development within particular areas. "Digital phenotyping," "ethics," "virtual reality," and "implementation science" emerge as niche themes by focalizing on deriving and assessing mental health metrics, ethical implications of AI, and therapy through immersive technologies. The presence of systematic review suggests increasing attention toward synthesizing evidence to evaluate the effectiveness of digital mental health solutions.

Emerging or declining themes (potential future trends or underdeveloped topics)
"Intervention" and "adherence" are clusters that emerge as themes indicating the suffering of research impacts derived from evaluating the effectiveness of digital mental health programs on various population groups. The emergence of "mobile health (mHealth)" and

"randomized controlled trials" indicates increased attention is being paid to the evidentiary based on the substantiation of the psychosocial software solutions in mental health. Furthermore, "digital interventions" and "implementation" suggest that attention is being paid to these interventions' actual use and practicality.

The research thematic trends (Figure 6.10) in the domain of digital mental health demonstrate an evolution from the general consideration of mental health topics to more focused discussions on digital interventions, marking shifts in research foci and the state of technology. At first, these studies were confined to the fundamental problems of mental health, such as depression, anxiety, and stress. With the rise of telehealth, AI, and various other digital health platforms, these themes gradually started integrating into digital platforms. Ethical concerns have been replaced with more sophisticated forms, such as digital phenotyping, which relies on AI for mental health evaluation to automate psychological evaluations. Digital intervention frameworks used to be the focus of general discussion, but now, such frameworks are increasingly used in psychotherapy and cognitive bias modification. The increasing importance placed on systematic reviews underscores the adoption of digital mental health interventions and emphasizes the need to assess their effectiveness.

In addition, the application of AI has grown considerably, as has digital phenotyping, helping to reinforce the diagnosis and treatment

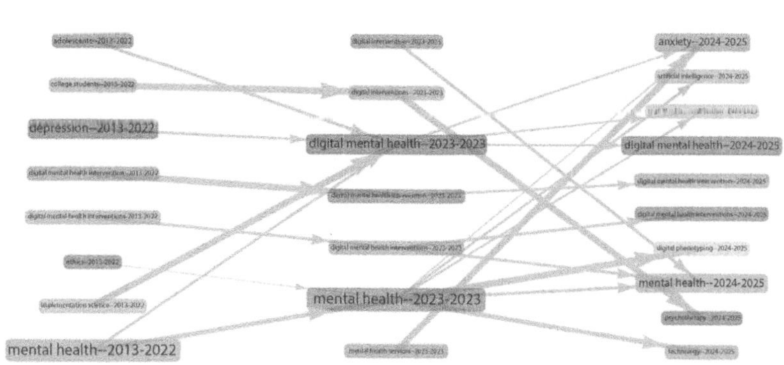

Figure 6.10 Thematic evolution. **Source:** Developed by the authors based on R.

of mental conditions using precise analytics, positioning these constructs as pillars of the domain. The fade from a research focus on depression into anxiety suggests changing priorities, particularly concerning adolescents. Furthermore, the framing of implementation science underscores the importance of ease of use and impact of digitally mediated interventions within real-life contexts. The evolution of digital mental health research has developed from general conversations about mental health concerns to a more focused, technological approach that prioritizes invention, efficiency, and the easy availability of mental health services.

6.5 Collaboration and Knowledge Dissemination

6.5.1 Collaboration Network

The examination of authorship partnerships (Figure 6.11) in the context of digital mental health research reveals an expanding cross-disciplinary collaboration network. Professionals from various disciplines, such as psychology, psychiatry, computer science, and public health, are beginning to work together to assess digital mental health interventions. The presence of strong collaboration clusters suggests the existence of powerful centers of innovation, particularly in AI, telehealth, and digital phenotyping. Some nascent connections point to the growth of international cooperation, abstracting the importance of information technology in mental health services. In addition, the network demonstrates a shift away from siloed research toward more cooperative and integrated frameworks that broaden knowledge transfer processes and streamline the advancement of efficient remote mental healthcare technologies.

The collaboration graph for the digital mental health research domain indicates that leading universities and research institutions across the globe have established strong partnerships. Harvard University, the University of Oxford, and the University of

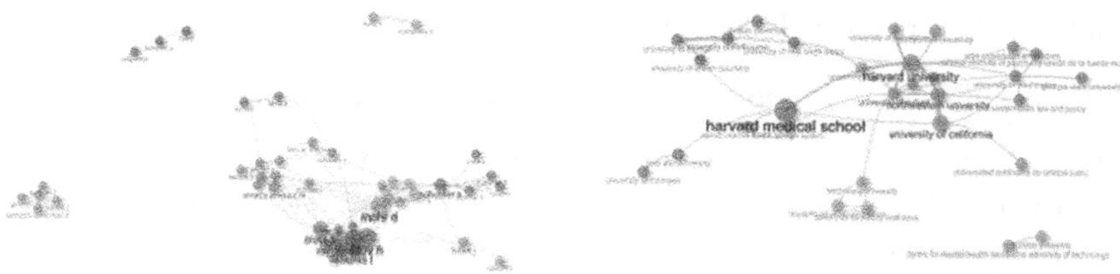

Figure 6.11 Authors and affiliation collaborations. **Source:** Developed by the authors based on R.

Washington are among the most influential and are central knowledge exchange hubs. Noteworthy universities from Australia, the United States, Canada, and Europe have made significant contributions that show the international scope of digital mental health research. Even though some institutions possess excellent connectivity and influence, others appear more solitary and disconnected. This suggests that those chains of institutions could be more actively engaged in cross-discipline or cross-border collaborations. Medical schools, alongside departments of neuroscience and specialized centers dealing with mental health issues, demonstrate the application of diverse resources to address mental health technological challenges.

6.6 Future Directions for a Digital Mental Health Ecosystem

Addressing issues with the integration of AI, user interaction, early intervention for adolescent mental health concerns, engagement monitoring using digital phenotyping, and enhancing the adaptability and impact of solutions within the healthcare system are some of the ways this set of research aims to advance the framework of the ecosystem of digital mental health.

Table 6.7 presents the key future research directions derived from this work, grouped by focus areas, objectives, and guiding research question.

Table 6.7 Future research directions.

Key area of focus	Objective	Research questions
Integration of artificial intelligence in digital mental health	Explore the possible use of AI in diagnosing, treating, and monitoring mental health disorders using digital channels.	1. What diagnostic and treatment standards of effectiveness can be improved with the incorporation of AI tools into digital mental health platforms?
		2. How does AI ethically intervene? AI tools raise ethical issues in mental health therapy, and how can this be solved?
User engagement and adherence in digital mental health interventions	To address sustained effectiveness through increased user engagement and adherence to digital mental health programs along with the maintenance of long-term sustainment.	1. What are the determinants of participation and sustained compliance among users in digital mental health interventions?
		2. In what ways can digital mental health programs be tailored in order to maximize user enrollment and minimize attrition?
Effectiveness of digital interventions for youth mental health	To address the use of digital mental health solutions among the youth population with regard to issues of anxiety and depression.	1. What are the impacts of mental health digital solutions among the youth population diagnosed with varying degrees of mental health disorders?
		2. Which digital mental health platforms are most popular with young users, and what accounts for their popularity?

(Continued)

Table 6.7 Future research directions. (*Continued*)

Key area of focus	Objective	Research questions
Digital phenotyping for mental health assessment	Investigate how mental health assessment and monitoring can be real-time and data-driven through the use of digital phenotyping technologies.	1. In what ways can digital phenotyping be applied for active monitoring and predicting mental health problems in real time?
		2. What are the data privacy and ethical issues of digital phenotyping in mental health research and practice?
Implementation science in digital mental health solutions	Evaluate the clinical and organizational factors that hinder or promote the scaling-up of digital interventions for mental health across different health system contexts.	1. What are the primary concerns regarding the execution of digital mental health services in various health systems?
		2. In what ways can implementation science enhance the effectiveness and enduring impact of digital mental health interventions?

Source: Developed by the authors.

6.7 Conclusion

This particular study investigates the new phenomenon of the digital mental health research ecosystem, which appeared during an episode of the COVID-19 pandemic and was subsequently accelerated by the progress of technology. A systematic review and bibliometric analysis conducted in accordance with PRISMA guidelines show that there has been a marked increase in research output since the year 2020, signaling increased interest in addressing mental health issues through technology. Citation patterns show that "old" studies continue to garner high citation counts, whereas "new" publications have yet to establish their full impact.

The key constitutive journals of the field include *JMIR Mental Health*, *JOCACP*, *FIP*, and *GFHJ*, which identifies the nexus between digital gaming and mental health. Leadership in this research area is predominantly American, with increasing input from New Zealand, Kenya, and Australia, reflecting the research field's global diversity. The impact is not uniformly distributed; some researchers dominate with a few highly influential studies, whereas others disseminate impact through many publications.

Thematic and keyword analyses reveal foundational research topics, which include depression, anxiety, mHealth, telehealth, and AI-driven interventions. A co-occurrence network also illustrates the strong interconnections between these topics, indicating a movement toward integrating technology into mental healthcare. Developing themes such as digital phenotyping, AI ethics, and virtual reality therapy signify a shift toward more data-centric approaches in evaluating and treating mental health issues. The focus has shifted from general debates concerning mental health to the development of targeted digital methods, especially AI and implementation science geared toward real-world problem-solving.

A three-field path analysis highlights the relationships between authors, keywords, and publication sources, illustrating the connections forming within disciplines in digital mental health. Clinical psychology, public health, and digital technology converge, highlighting the need for interdisciplinary collaboration. Insights from bibliometrics showcase the dynamic global research network and evolving thematic shifts alongside the multidisciplinary participation in the creation of a digitally comprehensive ecosystem of mental health.

International contributions alongside Myrick from the United States (Los Angeles County), Torous from Harvard Medical School, and Schueller from the University of California, Irvine, have significantly shaped the field. Focusing on the role of AI, telemedicine, and other digital health technologies as primary research areas is foundational to the interconnections themes. The emergence of digital phenotyping and ethical concerns showcases a shift toward sophisticated uses of AI and data.

Effective, scalable, and ethical technology-driven solutions require specialization around mental health, so interdisciplinary collaboration is essential. Thematic shift evolution emphasizes the growing focus on transforming digital solutions to integrated healthcare systems at scale. Diverse healthcare systems face advancements in optimizing mental health strategies, so continuous research, investments, and global partnerships are vital. A substantial impact toward building a comprehensive digital mental health ecosystem greatly relies on enhanced interdisciplinary collaboration.

6.8 Limitations

This chapter offers insights into the digital mental health research landscape, but several limitations must be discussed. Based on citation analysis, older studies continue to dominate citation counts. This phenomenon can potentially distort the impact of newer publications because old research requires a considerably more extended period as newer publications build up citations. This indicates that citation-based metrics alone may not represent the influence, however limited, of more recent studies. Moreover, the regional distribution of research parts poses another limitation. As the study has already discussed, the dominant contribution of the United States and other leading countries is significant; contributions from low- and middle-income countries may be seriously underestimated due to inequitable funding for research, subscription-based access to publication avenues, and poor inclusion in databases, which diminishes the generalizability of the findings to the broader world. To overcome these limitations, this study suggests refining the analytical focus on high-impact publications to be indexed in SSCI, ABDC, ABS, and FT 50, broadening data, enhancing impact assessment techniques, and integrating evaluation metrics. Despite the stated limitations, this study captures the scope of rapid acceleration and change of digital mental health research. Subsequent efforts need to shift toward comprehensively understanding innovations in digital mental health.

AI disclosure statement: The author acknowledges the use of AI-based tools for minor language editing or grammatical correction. However, all intellectual contributions, analyses, and conclusions presented in this chapter are entirely the author's own.

References

1. Balcombe, L. and De Leo, D., Digital mental health challenges and the horizon ahead for solutions. *JMIR Ment. Health*, *8*, 3, e26811, 2021.
2. Wies, B., Landers, C., Ienca, M., Digital mental health for young people: a scoping review of ethical promises and challenges. *Front. Digital Health*, *3*, 697072, 2021.
3. Altaf Dar, M., Maqbool, M., Ara, I., Zehravi, M., The intersection of technology and mental health: enhancing access and care. *Int. J. Adolesc. Med. Health*, *35*, 5, 423–428, 2023.
4. Naslund, J.A., Aschbrenner, K.A., Araya, R., Marsch, L.A., Unützer, J., Patel, V., Bartels, S.J., Digital technology for treating and preventing mental disorders in low-income and middle-income countries: A narrative review of the literature. *Lancet Psychiatry*, *4*, 6, 486–500, 2017.
5. Naslund, J.A., Gonsalves, P.P., Gruebner, O., Pendse, S.R., Smith, S.L., Sharma, A., Raviola, G., Digital innovations for global mental health: Opportunities for data science, task sharing, and early intervention. *Curr. Treat. Options Psychiatry*, *6*, 337–351, 2019.
6. Philippe, T.J., Sikder, N., Jackson, A., Koblanski, M.E., Liow, E., Pilarinos, A., Vasarhelyi, K., Digital health interventions for delivery of mental health care: Systematic and comprehensive meta-review. *JMIR Ment. Health*, *9*, 5, e35159, 2022.
7. Anjum, S., Ullah, R., Rana, M.S., Ali Khan, H., Memon, F.S., Ahmed, Y., Faryal, R., COVID-19 pandemic: A serious threat for public mental health globally. *Psychiatr. Danub.*, *32*, 2, 245–250, 2020.

8. Silove, D., Ventevogel, P., Rees, S., The contemporary refugee crisis: An overview of mental health challenges. *World Psychiatry*, *16*, 2, 130–139, 2017.
9. Lange, K.W., Coronavirus disease 2019 (COVID-19) and global mental health. *Global Health J.*, *5*, 1, 31–36, 2021.
10. Nochaiwong, S., Ruengorn, C., Thavorn, K., Hutton, B., Awiphan, R., Phosuya, C., Wongpakaran, T., Global prevalence of mental health issues among the general population during the coronavirus disease-2019 pandemic: a systematic review and meta-analysis. *Sci. Rep.*, *11*, 1, 10173, 2021.
11. Gureje, O., Nortje, G., Makanjuola, V., Oladeji, B.D., Seedat, S., Jenkins, R., The role of global traditional and complementary systems of medicine in the treatment of mental health disorders. *Lancet Psychiatry*, *2*, 2, 168–177, 2015.
12. Kennedy, J., Rhodes, K., Walls, C.A., Asplin, B.R., Access to emergency care: Restricted by long waiting times and cost and coverage concerns. *Ann. Emerg. Med.*, *43*, 5, 567–573, 2004.
13. Weissman, J.S., Stern, R., Fielding, S.L., Epstein, A.M., Delayed access to health care: Risk factors, reasons, and consequences, 1991.
14. Naiker, U., FitzGerald, G., Dulhunty, J.M., Rosemann, M., Time to wait: A systematic review of strategies that affect out-patient waiting times. *Aust. Health Rev.*, *42*, 3, 286–293, 2017.
15. Ansell, D., Crispo, J.A., Simard, B., Bjerre, L.M., Interventions to reduce wait times for primary care appointments: A systematic review. *BMC Health Serv. Res.*, *17*, 1–9, 2017.
16. Smith, K.A., Blease, C., Faurholt-Jepsen, M., Firth, J., Van Daele, T., Moreno, C., Cipriani, A., Digital mental health: Challenges and next steps. *BMJ Ment. Health*, *26*, 1, 2023.
17. Malik, A., Technology and Mental Health: Harnessing Digital Interventions for Support and Treatment. *J. Psychol. Health Soc. Chall.*, *1*, 02, 149–162, 2023.
18. Thirupathi, L., Kaashipaka, V., Dhanaraju, M., Katakam, V., AI and IoT in Mental Health Care: From Digital Diagnostics to Personalized, Continuous Support, in: *Intelligent Systems and IoT Applications in Clinical Health*, pp. 271–294, IGI Global, Hershey, Pennsylvania, USA, 2025.
19. Torous, J., Larsen, M.E., Depp, C., Cosco, T.D., Barnett, I., Nock, M.K., Firth, J., Smartphones, sensors, and machine learning to advance

real-time prediction and interventions for suicide prevention: A review of current progress and next steps. *Curr. Psychiatry Rep.*, *20*, 1–6, 2018.
20. Rostami, M., Abdi, M., Asadi, N.Z., Predicting the Future of Mental Health Interventions: The Role of Digital Therapeutics. *J. Foresight Public Health*, *2*, 2, 33–51, 2025.
21. O'Daffer, A., Colt, S.F., Wasil, A.R., Lau, N., Efficacy and conflicts of interest in randomized controlled trials evaluating Headspace and Calm apps: Systematic review. *JMIR Ment. Health*, *9*, 9, e40924, 2022.
22. Pavlopoulos, A., Rachiotis, T., Maglogiannis, I., An overview of tools and technologies for anxiety and depression management using AI. *Appl. Sci.*, *14*, 19, 9068, 2024.
23. Nelson, J., Kaplan, J., Simerly, G., Nutter, N., Edson-Heussi, A., Woodham, B., Broman-Fulks, J., The balance and integration of artificial intelligence within cognitive behavioral therapy interventions. *Curr. Psychol.*, 1–11, 2025.
24. Jo, E., Kouaho, W.J., Schueller, S.M., Epstein, D.A., Exploring user perspectives of and ethical experiences with teletherapy apps: Qualitative analysis of user reviews. *JMIR Ment. Health*, *10*, e49684, 2023.
25. Delawalla, C.N. and Lorenzo-Luaces, L., "Better" Help? Ethical Considerations for Therapists Using Telehealth Matching Platforms, 2024.
26. Hebbar, S. and Vandana, B., Artificial Intelligence in Future Telepsychiatry and Psychotherapy for E-Mental Health Revolution, in: *Computational Intelligence in Medical Decision Making and Diagnosis*, pp. 39–60, CRC Press, Boca Raton, FL, USA, 2023.
27. Gkintoni, E., Vassilopoulos, S.P., Nikolaou, G., Next-Generation Cognitive-Behavioral Therapy for Depression: Integrating Digital Tools, Teletherapy, and Personalization for Enhanced Mental Health Outcomes. *Medicina*, *61*, 3, 431, 2025.
28. Golinelli, D., Boetto, E., Carullo, G., Nuzzolese, A.G., Landini, M.P., Fantini, M.P., Adoption of digital technologies in health care during the COVID-19 pandemic: Systematic review of early scientific literature. *J. Med. Internet Res.*, *22*, 11, e22280, 2020.
29. Luo, J., Tong, L., Crotty, B.H., Somai, M., Taylor, B., Osinski, K., George, B., Telemedicine adoption during the COVID-19 pandemic: Gaps and inequalities. *Appl. Clin. Inf.*, *12*, 04, 836–844, 2021.

30. Chang, J.E., Lai, A.Y., Gupta, A., Nguyen, A.M., Berry, C.A., Shelley, D.R., Rapid transition to telehealth and the digital divide: Implications for primary care access and equity in a post-COVID era. *Milbank Q.*, *99*, 2, 340–368, 2021.
31. Anikwe, C.V., Nweke, H.F., Ikegwu, A.C., Egwuonwu, C.A., Onu, F.U., Alo, U.R., Teh, Y.W., Mobile and wearable sensors for data-driven health monitoring system: State-of-the-art and future prospect. *Expert Syst. Appl.*, *202*, 117362, 2022.
32. Moher, D., Liberati, A., Tetzlaff, J., Altman, D.G., Preferred reporting items for systematic reviews and meta-analyses: The PRISMA statement. *BMJ*, *339*, 2009.
33. Donthu, N., Kumar, S., Mukherjee, D., Pandey, N., Lim, W.M., How to conduct a bibliometric analysis: An overview and guidelines. *J. Bus. Res.*, *133*, 285–296, 2021.
34. Ellegaard, O. and Wallin, J.A., The bibliometric analysis of scholarly production: How great is the impact? *Scientometrics*, *105*, 1809–1831, 2015.
35. Pati, D. and Lorusso, L.N., How to write a systematic review of the literature. *HERD: Health Environ. Res. Des. J.*, *11*, 1, 15–30, 2018.
36. Sauer, P.C. and Seuring, S., How to conduct systematic literature reviews in management research: A guide in 6 steps and 14 decisions. *Rev. Managerial Sci.*, *17*, 5, 1899–1933, 2023.
37. Zhu, J. and Liu, W., A tale of two databases: the use of Web of Science and Scopus in academic papers. *Scientometrics*, *123*, 1, 321–335, 2020.
38. Kumpulainen, M. and Seppänen, M., Combining Web of Science and Scopus datasets in citation-based literature study. *Scientometrics*, *127*, 10, 5613–5631, 2022.
39. Torous, J., Myrick, K.J., Rauseo-Ricupero, N., Firth, J., Digital mental health and COVID-19: Using technology today to accelerate the curve on access and quality tomorrow. *JMIR Ment. Health*, *7*, 3, e18848, 2020.
40. Schueller, S.M., Hunter, J.F., Figueroa, C., Aguilera, A., Use of digital mental health for marginalized and underserved populations. *Curr. Treat. Options Psychiatry*, 6, 243–255, 2019.
41. Graham, A.K., Lattie, E.G., Powell, B.J., Lyon, A.R., Smith, J.D., Schueller, S.M., Mohr, D.C., Implementation strategies for digital mental health interventions in health care settings. *Am. Psychol.*, *75*, 8, 1080, 2020.

42. Schueller, S.M. and Torous, J., Scaling evidence-based treatments through digital mental health. *Am. Psychol.*, *75*, 8, 1093, 2020.
43. Lattie, E.G., Schueller, S.M., Sargent, E., Stiles-Shields, C., Tomasino, K.N., Corden, M.E., Mohr, D.C., Uptake and usage of IntelliCare: A publicly available suite of mental health and well-being apps. *Internet Interv.*, *4*, 152–158, 2016.
44. Pine, R., Fleming, T., McCallum, S., Sutcliffe, K., The effects of casual videogames on anxiety, depression, stress, and low mood: A systematic review. *Games Health J.*, *9*, 4, 255–264, 2020.
45. Osborn, T.L., Rodriguez, M., Wasil, A.R., Venturo-Conerly, K.E., Gan, J., Alemu, R.G., Weisz, J.R., Single-session digital intervention for adolescent depression, anxiety, and well-being: Outcomes of a randomized controlled trial with Kenyan adolescents. *J. Consult. Clin. Psychol.*, *88*, 7, 657, 2020.
46. Parker, L., Halter, V., Karliychuk, T., Grundy, Q., How private is your mental health app data? An empirical study of mental health app privacy policies and practices. *Int. J. Law Psychiatry*, *64*, 198–204, 2019.
47. Wasil, A.R., Gillespie, S., Patel, R., Petre, A., Venturo-Conerly, K.E., Shingleton, R.M., DeRubeis, R.J., Reassessing evidence-based content in popular smartphone apps for depression and anxiety: Developing and applying user-adjusted analyses. *J. Consult. Clin. Psychol.*, *88*, 11, 983, 2020.

7

Digital Psychiatry: Foundations and Innovations Driving the PsyTech Revolution in Mental Healthcare

Galiveeti Poornima[1]*, Sukruth Gowda M.A.[2] and Y. Mohamadi Begum[1]

[1]School of Engineering and Technology, S-Vyasa Deemed to be University, Bangalore, India
[2]Department of AI, SVIT, Bangalore, India

Abstract
Digital psychiatry is an emerging paradigm that marries digital technologies to traditional psychiatric care. This chapter covers some of the early work underlying digital psychiatry and its role in the envelope of a new PsyTech revolution. Various technologies, including telepsychiatry, mobile health applications, wearable devices, artificial intelligence, virtual reality, and digital phenotyping, are discussed, among others, for their potential to transform the diagnosis, treatment, monitoring, and prevention of mental health disorders. The chapter outlines the fundamental ideas of this new paradigm, including the importance of interdisciplinary collaboration, patient-centered treatments, and ethical issues. It draws attention to the many advantages, such as improved access, individualized treatment, and scalability, as well as the drawbacks, such as data privacy issues, regulatory obstacles, and the digital divide. This chapter presents a vision for how mental healthcare delivery might operate moving forward through the lens of real-world case studies and emerging trends. It illustrates how technology can both create new solutions while addressing barriers to care. It urges that politicians, technologists, and doctors work together to shape what psychiatry looks like in the digital age.

***Keywords*:** Digital psychiatry, artificial intelligence in mental health, telepsychiatry, mental health technologies, digital phenotyping, digital therapeutics, smart mental health monitoring

**Corresponding author*: varaprabha.lita@gmail.com

Raghavendra M. Devadas, Vani Hiremani, Preethi, Praveen Gujjar, Sapna R. and Manoj Shettar (eds.) Psychiatry and Technology, (195–254) © 2026 Scrivener Publishing LLC

7.1 Introduction

Digital psychiatry offers longitudinal tracking and individualized behavioral therapeutic tools that diverge from the collective norms that dominate most psychiatric practices to derive the clinical encounter from self to disclosed symptoms. Digital psychiatry is an evolving transdisciplinary field that integrates technology into psychiatry with the potential to add value to diagnosis, treatment, and management of psychiatric diseases [1]. This multidimensional perspective holds largely untapped knowledge and potential for implementation of near real-time, precise mental health status reporting, artificial intelligence (AI), mobile health (mHealth), and wearable biosensors, as well as digital therapeutics (DTx) in this area.

In fact, in addition to its clinical practice implications, digital psychiatry must be considered in relation to public health [2, 3], workplace mental health [3], and education [3]. By targeting underserved populations, mental health chatbots, telepsychiatry platforms, and smartphone-based cognitive behavioral therapy (CBT) apps have democratized mental healthcare [4] with critical implications for individuals living in remote and rural areas, where psychiatric resources are limited. These solutions offer a sanctuary for emotional support and lower stigma surrounding the matter because therapeutic tools can be utilized by users in private and confidentially, empowering individuals to ask for support from others without being concerned about being judged [5].

Digital psychiatry offers many opportunities but also presents challenges regarding data privacy ethics and regulation [6]. Using AI technologies for diagnostics and predictive modeling raises issues of algorithmic bias, accuracy, and clinical accountability [7]. Furthermore, the increasing dependence on the digital platform requires strong infrastructure for security standards, seamless interface, and ethical data governance [8]. Thus, we must establish limits to synchronize the rapid movement of technology with the guiding principles of psychiatry without losing sight of the patient at the heart of the matter.

7.1.1 The Evolving Role of Technology in Mental Health

The mental healthcare sector has undergone a complete transition through DTx. Long waiting lists, geographical hindrances, and a scarcity of mental health professionals impede traditional psychiatric services [9]. In response to the mental health crisis, various digital tools have been used to improve traditional treatments, such as telepsychiatry, AI-assisted mental health evaluations, and digital phenotyping [10]. The introduction of telepsychiatry allows for arrangements of consultation to be made through video conferencing, eliminating geographical and logistical barriers and ensuring that mental health doctors are available when patients require them [11].

Application of AI in medical image analysis, diagnosis, and electronic medical records and AI dominance in various sectors: Healthcare is one of the sectors that have been extensively impacted by AI presiding over the organization of patient data, record keeping, and information retrieval [12]. Deep learning networks trained on large datasets can recognize fragmented profiles of depression, anxiety, and schizophrenia that would otherwise go unnoticed in the traditional clinical setting [13]. Such prediction helps identify lifestyle-related risk factors early, enabling timely intervention before mental health symptoms worsen [14]. Wearable devices (e.g., smartwatches, electroencephalogram [EEG] headsets) that continuously monitor biometric data can also provide information about sleep condition, stress levels, and emotional state, thus allowing for individualized treatment [15].

Another critical aspect of technology's importance in psychiatry is its capacity to support scalable and self-directed interventions [16]. Mobile applications providing guided meditation, mood tracking, and AI-assisted therapy have enabled individuals to take control of their mental well-being. In addition, virtual reality (VR) and augmented reality (AR) are integrated into therapeutic sessions for the treatment of phobias, posttraumatic stress disorder (PTSD), anxiety disorders, and others [17]. By simulating controlled environments, these technologies enable patients to face their fears and begin working through them in a safe space.

Nonetheless, with the speedy transition of mental healthcare to a digital platform, ethical oversight and responsible novel innovation are needed moving forward [18]. If digital psychiatry does seem to be an effectual path to pursue as its adoption increases, aspects such as data privacy, technology dependence, and the spread of disinformation will need to be mitigated to make sure that mental health treatment through a human-centered lens rather than as it eventually becomes, as a supplement or replacement through the raw numbers of mental health treatment [19]. Although psychiatric digital innovation offers exciting potential, it needs to develop responsibly, ensuring clinical utility, safety for patients, and ethical adherence.

7.1.2 Objectives and Scope of the Chapter

The purpose of this chapter is to give an overview of digital psychiatry, from its origins through technological advances and steps going forward. This chapter explores how technology and psychiatry converge, examining some of the core questions around the use, effectiveness, and ethics of technology in mental health. The goal is to create a happy medium that combines the best of both worlds, so that digital treatments supplement rather than supplant patient-centered therapy.

In its first portion, it focuses on the history and theory of digital psychiatry, describing the ongoing history of technology and mental health and how some of the ideas that built digital psychiatry took shape during that history. You will discuss how big data analytics, wearable technology, and AI-enabled diagnostics are transforming psychiatric research and treatment protocols. Our journey will explore the ethical implications, such as data privacy, informed consent, and algorithmic bias, highlighting the need for responsible digital mental health development.

The next section will review new technologies and their application in psychiatry. If you would like to discuss this subject in greater detail, a study will be made to examine AI influence on mental health diagnostics, increasing telepsychiatry use, and digital pharmaceutical impact in behavior therapy. To illustrate how they can change psychiatric solutions, we will explore emerging applications such as VR-based therapy, blockchain-facilitated health data management, and wearable biosensors for real-time updates on mood and mood shifts.

Lastly, the upcoming challenges, limits, and mechanical aspects of digital psychiatry will be discussed. It will address regulatory hurdles, cybersecurity challenges, and the urgent need for standardized clinical validation of digital tools. The final part will encounter future developments of the PsyTech revolution including brain–computer interfaces (BCIs), quantum computing applied to the research of mental health, and improved psychiatry through AI. This chapter will address these issues and more by discussing technology and psychiatric care from several angles, so that we may learn how to best implement mental health services for wide populations that are lacking access. Figure 7.1 illustrates the digital psychiatry ecosystem and its interlinked technological components.

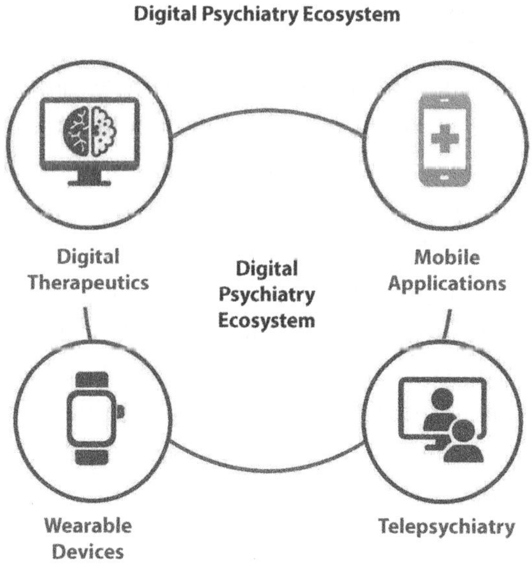

Figure 7.1 Digital psychiatry ecosystem.

7.2 Foundations of Digital Psychiatry

The future of digital psychiatry and its barriers and challenges will be discussed. It will look at legislative challenges, cybersecurity threats, and the critical need for standardized clinical validation processes for digital tools. The final part will look into possible future trends in the PsyTech revolution, including BCIs, quantum computing for probing the mind, and AI-hyperaged precision psychiatry. This chapter aims to similarly provide a framework for utilizing technology-enabled psychiatric interventions to mitigate mental health treatment inequities that are similarly stark in marginalized communities.

During the 1990s and early 2000s, internet-based interventions and computerized CBT programs expanded the field of digital psychiatry [22]. New ways for persons to access mental health resources emerged (e.g., through websites providing self-help modules, psycho education and online forums) without the barriers of attending physical appointments [23]. Telemedicine and telepsychiatry have transformed the way psychiatric care is delivered, allowing remote consultations and therapy sessions through video conferencing. These advances are particularly useful for rural and underserved communities with limited access to mental health professionals [11].

The 2010s marked the AI and data-driven revolution in psychiatry, with machine learning models being applied to analyze patient data, predict mental health disorders, and personalize treatment plans [24]. Advances in wearable technology, smartphone-based mood tracking, and digital biomarkers introduced continuous mental health monitoring, allowing real-time assessment of behavioral and physiological indicators such as sleep patterns, heart rate variability (HRV), and voice modulation [25]. The integration of VR and AR into psychiatric therapy also became a significant breakthrough, offering exposure therapy, PTSD treatment, and anxiety management in immersive virtual environments [17].

Today, digital psychiatry is rapidly evolving with the advent of blockchain for secure health data management, generative AI for mental health chatbots, and neurotechnology for BCIs [26]. The field continues

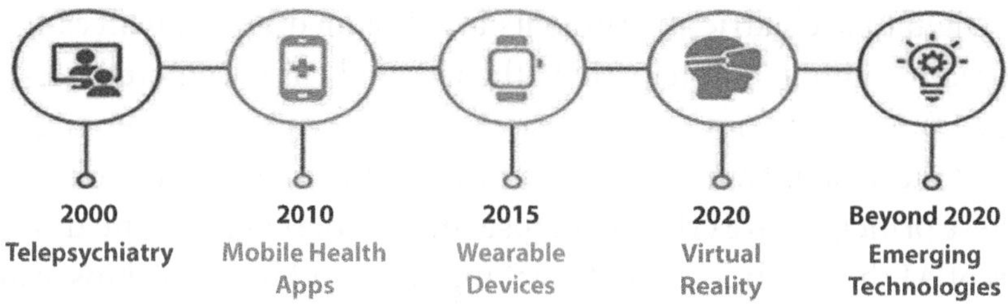

Figure 7.2 Evolution timeline of digital psychiatry.

to push boundaries, aiming to bridge the gap between traditional psychiatric practice and precision psychiatry—a personalized approach to mental healthcare driven by big data analytics and AI. Nonetheless, these advancements in digital psychiatry are not without their ethical, regulatory, and clinical challenges, which will need to be overcome if these innovations are to be scientifically validated, ethically applied, and readily available [27]. Figure 7.2 presents the evolution timeline of digital psychiatry across major technological milestones.

7.2.1 Theoretical Frameworks and Principles Guiding Digital Mental Health

Digital psychiatry is informed by a number of theoretical models and principles that guide its development, implementation, and evaluation [20]. One holds a biopsychosocial model [28] as a basic theoretical scaffold that helps to amalgamate the biological, psychological, and social factors involved in the understanding of mental health disorders. Then, this has been further expanded to include digital biomarkers, algorithm-driven psychological assessments, other data such as social media behaviors, etc., adding to the overall picture of a comprehensive digital psychiatry picture of your mental status.

CBT is a fundamental pillar of most mobile mental health applications, AI-based therapy programs, and self-guided interventions [30]. Digital CBT cohorts provide structured exercises, automated feedback, and real-time cognitive restructuring techniques to help clients work through depression, anxiety, and PTSD. The efficacy of digital CBT is well proven, and in numerous cases, research has shown outcomes equivalent to—or better than—face-to-face therapy.

Digital psychiatric instruments are designed on Influences from human–computer interaction theory and user-centered design (UCD) methodology [31]. These strategies emphasize user engagement, accessibility, and usability of digital mental health solutions. These principles are critical because they enable engagement: designers of AI therapy bots, mood-tracking apps, and wearable biosensors build intuitive and response interventions that adapt to the realities of care in a way that is culturally accessible and therefore maximizes patient adherence and overall effectiveness of digital intervention.

A complementary model with theoretical implications for the conforming of digital psychiatry is the scientific model of digital phenotyping, which calls for contiguous "real-world" collection of behavioral and physiological data captured through smartphones and wearables to extract patterns of prevalence that characterize mental health. This approach uses machine learning to analyze data points such as typing speed, vocal tone, social media activity, and sleep patterns to determine early signs of mental problems. Although the digital phenotype holds great potential for preemptive intervention, it raises issues of privacy and permission, as well as data ethics, given the rapid pace with which technology has developed; this highlights the need for a balance between technological advancement and human rights.

On the contrary, a complementary model that can clarify the theory behind digital psychiatry is digital phenotyping as a science framework that encourages gathering real-time behavioral and physiological data through smartphones and wearables to detect patterns of common mental health. This methodology provides an automated approach in which machine learning analyzes individual data points including typing speed, vocal inflection, social media usage, and sleep patterns to determine early signs of potential mental health disorders. The digital phenotype certainly holds a lot of promise for early intervention; however, it also raises some critical issues surrounding privacy, consent, and the ethics of data usage that transcends technology, requiring balance between technology and human being rights.

7.2.2 Ethical, Legal, and Privacy Considerations in Digital Psychiatric Interventions

As it evolves, it will pose serious ethical, legal, and privacy challenges. The main concern is data privacy and security, given that digital mental health platforms can collect large volumes of sensitive personal data [34]. Applications for mHealth, artificial intelligence assessment for mental health, or telepsychiatry systems gather data on the behavioral patterns of clients, physiological parameters, or speech patterns, which, in turn, can lead to data leaks or loss, unauthorized access, and misuse by third parties [35]. User confidence and ethical integrity in digital psychiatry heavily depend on end-to-end encryption, informed consent, and regulatory compliance [36]. Table 7.1 summarizes global data protection laws and frameworks relevant to digital psychiatric practices.

Table 7.1 Overview of data governance regulations relevant to digital psychiatry.

Framework	Jurisdiction	Focus areas	Compliance tools	Limitations
HIPAA	USA	Health data privacy and security	Encryption, Access logs	Does not address AI bias
GDPR	EU	Data protection, consent	Consent forms, audit	Cross-border complexity
MHCA	India	Mental healthcare delivery rights	Digital consent, record	Vague on digital tools
AI Bill of Rights	Global (proposed)	Ethical AI use in healthcare	Fairness, transparency	Not yet fully enforced
FDA guidelines	USA	Digital therapeutics and devices	Clinical validation	Lengthy approval timelines

A significant ethical dilemma is algorithmic bias and fairness. The AI models used in digital psychiatry depend on datasets that may insufficiently represent varied populations. This may result in skewed predictions, perhaps leading to misdiagnoses or diminished efficacy among specific demographic groups, particularly underprivileged communities. Addressing these biases necessitates transparent AI development, varied data representation, and ongoing auditing of machine learning models to provide equitable and inclusive mental health evaluations.

The legal environment for digital psychiatry is still being established with various legislations. Whereas several countries have implemented criteria for telemedicine interaction, encompassing data protection (e.g., General Data Protection Regulation [GDPR], Health Insurance Portability and Accountability Act [HIPAA]) and AI in healthcare, others do not possess explicit policies governing digital mental health technologies. Such frameworks must also delineate the explicit obligations of developers, healthcare professionals, and politicians in guaranteeing the ethical implementation of AI-driven psychiatric solutions [40].

Furthermore, the human experience of psychiatric recovery must be validated by a technology-mediated algorithm. Although digital psychiatry enhances accessibility and facilitates early diagnosis, it ought to complement, rather than replace, human-centered mental healthcare [41]. In the integration of AI-driven tools into psychiatry, ethical guidelines must emphasize the need of clinical oversight, patient autonomy, and informed permission [42]. Reconciling technical developments with human empathy will remain a significant problem in the digital transformation of psychiatry [43].

Digital psychiatry is grounded in its historical evolution, theoretical foundations, and ethical considerations. The evolution from early chatbot therapies to contemporary AI-driven diagnostics and wearable mental health monitoring has been significant. Digital psychiatry is the implementation of models of psychiatric care implementing widely utilized psychiatric constructs, behavioral frameworks, and UCD principles to drive individualized, data-informed mental healthcare. Significant ethical and legal frameworks will be needed as technology evolves to address equity, privacy, and inclusion. Understanding of these basics is critical for prudent and sustainable implementation of digital solutions in psychiatry.

7.3 Technological Innovations in Digital Psychiatry

Recent advances in technology, whether it be in diagnosis, therapy, or patient participation, have advanced psychiatry to new heights. The world of traditional psychiatric therapy has completely transformed into data-driven, customized, and widely available therapy using innovative technologies including so-called AI, wearables, mHealth, VR, and blockchain. In this section, we will explore the recent innovations that have been driving digital psychiatry and their potential impact and implications for mental healthcare.

7.3.1 AI and Machine Learning

AI technologies can revolutionize psychiatry aspects, mainly psychiatric diagnostics and predictive analytics, as they can enable physicians to facilitate more widespread detection of mental health illnesses more efficiently and accurately through pattern recognition and automation [29], enabling AI systems to tap into speech patterns, facial cues, social media activity, and other biometric information for the diagnosis of mental health disorders.

Machine learning algorithms then analyze large datasets to identify patterns that can predict the emergence of psychiatric illnesses, allowing for early treatment and intervention before symptoms worsen [45]. It is AI-powered natural language processing (NLP) applications that evaluate tone, diction, and fluency changes to detect cognitive decline or a psychological discomfort of a patient. Furthermore, the AI-driven study of neuroimaging points out some biomarkers related to psychiatric diseases, this clarifying the neurophysiological basis of psychiatric illness [46].

Mental health chatbots enabled by AI embedded in virtual therapist systems offer a rapid, scalable, widely accessible, and cost-effective method of deploying mental health treatment services [13]. These AI-powered solutions proffer personalized mental health therapies with the utilization of CBT principles, emotion identification, and adaptive learning.

Nearly all platforms concentrate on conversational therapy, mood monitoring, and cognitive restructuring exercises through services such as Woebot, Wysa, and Replikant [47]. These chatbots use a humanistic methodology to aid individuals in mitigating stress, anxiety, and depression by offering immediate coping strategies and therapeutic guidance. Virtual therapists may not completely supplant human therapists, although they serve as an essential conduit for individuals unable to access mental healthcare promptly.

Nonetheless, technological improvements in AI psychiatric care present ethical hurdles, including potential bias in AI models, data privacy issues, and the requirement for human monitoring. A bright future for AI in digital psychiatry may entail hybrid models that integrate AI-generated insights with human clinical judgment, ensuring that technology serves as a complement rather than a replacement for professional care.

7.3.2 Wearable Technology and Internet of Things in Mental Health

Wearable devices, combined with smartwatch devices, EEG headsets, biosensors, etc., continue to enhance mental health and well-being by collecting data continuously related to HRV, sleep, physical activity, and stress levels [48]. These data points offer vital insights into a patient's mental state and emotional health, enabling clinicians to identify early warning signs of anxiety, depression, or psychotic episodes. Selection of smart technology: Fitness trackers (e.g., Fitbit, Apple Watch, Oura Ring) monitor sleep quality and physical activity, which are associated with mental health conditions [49]. Alterations in sleep and fluctuations in heart rate can predict mood swings in individuals with bipolar disorder [50]. Similarly, neurofeedback wearables that use EEG monitor brainwave activity and can aid those suffering from conditions such as attention-deficit/hyperactivity disorder, PTSD, and generalized anxiety disorder [51].

Internet of Things (IoT)–enabled wearables can help to monitor patients' physiology and behavior in real time and hold potential for clinician to design personalized treatment based on daily variation in afflicted individual. By continuously keeping track of key mental health parameters, wearables can provide them with timely triggers for the intake of medicine, mindfulness or relaxation practices.

Through real-time feedbacks, AI-driven analytics improves personalization as it adapts therapeutic propositions that ease a dynamic approach to care. For example, when a wearable confirms that a user is in acute stress, they can receive breathing exercises, guided meditations, or approaches based on cognitive restructuring [53]. These modalities help patients in developing improved self-awareness, and improve self-regulation leading to an increase in treatment adherence and outcomes.

Still, the rapid advances have stirred worries about data security, the reliability of wearable sensor technology, and the morality of perpetual surveillance. Creative tactics such as supporting patient-centric data governance laws are key to building patient trust and preventing fines.

7.3.3 mHealth and Telepsychiatry

Wearables and IoT technology, when interlaced, offers a real-time analysis of patient data by their daily physiological and behavioral patterns, enabling the clinician to modify/manage treatment accordingly. Wearables are capable of monitoring mental health vital signs over time to provide on-demand interventions, including reminders to take medication, guided mindfulness, or relaxation techniques [50].

AI-powered analytics are capable of making suggestions that personalize therapy according to real-time input [54]. For example, when a wearable device detects that a user is stressed or about to panic, it could recommend breathing exercises, guided meditation, or cognitive restructuring techniques. Many of these therapies, which promote self-awareness and self-regulation skills, correlate with enhanced treatment adherence and outcomes for patients.

However, challenges remain including data security, the accuracy of wearable sensors, and ethical issues surrounding constant monitoring of patients. Therefore, to obtain patient confidence and compliance, transparent and end-user–centered data governance policies need to be enforced [55].

Telepsychiatry has significantly expanded access to mental healthcare, particularly for underserved and remote communities. Secure video conferencing technologies enhance the accessibility, affordability, and convenience of psychiatric care for patients.

Nonetheless, telepsychiatry presents several problems, including technological obstacles, digital literacy deficiencies, and regulatory issues. Ensuring data integrity against security vulnerabilities while providing privacy and equitable access to information addresses prevalent concerns. Moreover, specific health issues necessitate in-person assessment and treatment, which cannot be adequately addressed with contemporary virtual care. Addressing these difficulties will involve the advancement of telepsychiatry legislation, AI-enhanced diagnostics, and cohesive digital health solutions both within and beyond clinical practice.

7.3.4 VR/AR in Mental Health Interventions

VR and AR technologies are utilized in exposure treatment, mindfulness training, and stress management [57]. VR therapy allow patients to confront phobias, PTSD triggers, and social anxiety inside controlled, immersive settings.

For instance, VR exposure therapy has been effectively used for combat veterans with PTSD, enabling patients to progressively address horrific memories in a secure and structured environment [58]. Likewise, mindfulness applications such as TRIPP and Healium utilize VR to generate soothing, contemplative experiences that enhance relaxation and emotional control [59].

Psychiatric therapies are enhanced by VR and AR by improving sensory engagement and fostering emotional connections. Individuals with acute anxiety or depression frequently struggle to participate in traditional talk therapy; immersive VR sessions provide additional therapeutic avenues that promote calm and self-reflection [61].

Barriers include elevated expenses, restricted accessibility, and the potential for excessive dependence on virtual solutions. The decreasing cost and enhanced accessibility of VR/AR technology will certainly lead to a significant rise in its integration into routine psychiatric care.

7.3.5 Blockchain and Data Security in Digital Psychiatry

With the rise of AI-driven digital mental health solutions, data privacy and security have become major concerns. Blockchain technology offers a decentralized, tamper-proof system for storing and managing sensitive mental health data [62]. By using smart contracts and encrypted transactions, blockchain ensures secure access to patient records while preventing unauthorized data breaches.

Blockchain-powered electronic health records (EHRs) give patients greater control over their psychiatric history, allowing them to share data securely with selected providers [63]. This prevents misuse of sensitive information and enhances trust between patients and digital psychiatry platforms.

Despite its promise, blockchain in psychiatry faces scalability issues, regulatory hurdles, and the need for widespread adoption [64]. Addressing these challenges will require collaboration between technologists, psychiatrists, and policymakers to ensure secure and ethical implementation.

Technological innovations are reshaping psychiatry by making mental healthcare more accessible, personalized, and data-driven. Although AI, wearables, mHealth, VR, and blockchain offer groundbreaking opportunities, addressing ethical, regulatory, and implementation challenges will be essential for ensuring their sustainable integration into psychiatric care. Table 7.2 provides a comparative

Table 7.2 Comparison of emerging digital psychiatry technologies and their clinical applications.

Technology	Purpose	Example tools	Clinical use	Challenges
AI and ML	Diagnosis and prediction	Woebot, Wysa	Depression, anxiety	Bias, explainability
Wearables	Real-time monitoring	Fitbit, Muse	Sleep, mood, stress	Data reliability
Telepsychiatry	Remote consultation	Doxy.me, Amwell	Rural care, scheduling	Digital literacy
VR/AR	Immersive therapy	TRIPP, Healium	PTSD, phobias, anxiety	Cost, accessibility
Blockchain	Secure health records	Medicalchain	Data protection	Scalability, regulation

overview of major digital tools, their applications, and challenges in mental healthcare.

7.4 Core Principles of Digital Psychiatry

Digital psychiatry operates at the intersection of technology and mental health, bringing forth innovative solutions that improve accessibility, diagnostics, and treatment outcomes [65]. However, as these technologies evolve, it is essential to uphold core principles that ensure ethical, equitable, and patient-centered mental healthcare. This section explores three fundamental principles: ethical considerations, equity and accessibility, and patient-centered approaches.

7.4.1 Ethical Considerations (Privacy, Consent, and Security)

One of the most pressing ethical concerns in digital psychiatry is data privacy and security. Digital mental health platforms, AI-driven assessments, and wearable devices collect highly sensitive information, including biometric signals, behavioral patterns, and psychological responses [66]. Without stringent safeguards, these data can be vulnerable to breaches, misuse, or unauthorized access. The integrity of transmitted data must be guaranteed *via* end-to-end encryption, rigorous access restrictions, and compliance with healthcare information regulations, including HIPAA and the GDPR [67].

An additional crucial element is informed consent. An increasing quantity of these digital psychiatry tools is passive, signifying that they collect data *via* interactions with smartphones, social media activities, or physiological monitoring [25]. Users must be thoroughly apprised of the data being collected, the rationale behind it, and their choices to decline such acquisition. Ethical digital psychiatry solutions necessitate transparent data regulations, user-friendly permission methods, and real-time control over data-sharing preferences.

This extends beyond privacy; the ethical application of AI in mental care is a burgeoning topic. AI-driven mental health assessments and chatbots should avoid algorithmic bias, which can lead to misdiagnosis or discrimination against certain demographic groups. To uphold fairness, AI models must be trained on diverse, representative datasets and continuously audited for bias and accuracy.

7.4.2 Equity and Accessibility in Technology Deployment

Digital psychiatry has the potential to expand mental health access to underserved populations, but it also risks exacerbating health inequities if not deployed thoughtfully [68]. The digital divide—the gap between those with access to technology and those without—remains a significant challenge, particularly in low-income, rural, and marginalized communities [69]. Many mental health apps and telepsychiatry services require high-speed internet, smartphones, and digital literacy, which are not universally available [11].

To promote equitable mental healthcare, digital psychiatry initiatives must focus on inclusive design by:

- Developing low-bandwidth, offline-capable mental health apps for regions with limited internet access.

- Offering multilanguage support and culturally relevant content to ensure accessibility across diverse populations.
- Providing affordable or subsidized digital mental health services for economically disadvantaged individuals.

AI-driven psychiatric tools must be inclusive and fair, ensuring they work effectively across different ethnic, gender, and socioeconomic groups [70]. Many AI models in psychiatry are trained on datasets primarily derived from WEIRD (Western, educated, industrialized, rich, and democratic) populations, leading to biased outcomes when applied to other demographics [71].

Ensuring equity in digital psychiatry requires:

- Diverse data representation in AI training models to account for cultural and demographic differences.
- Bias mitigation techniques to reduce discriminatory patterns in AI-driven diagnoses.
- Regulatory oversight and ethical AI development to ensure fairness in mental health technology.

If these challenges are addressed, digital psychiatry has the real potential to solve its promise of wider access to high-quality mental healthcare to everyone, irrespective of socioeconomic background or geographical location.

7.4.3 Patient-Centered Approaches

Preferring for digital psychiatry solutions over the one-size-fits-all model described above, a patient-centered approach guarantees that the needs of individuals are addressed rather than the needs of a population as a whole [72]. So, personalized mental healthcare is important, because psychiatric disorders are highly complex and unique to each individual [73].

Thirupathi [66], accentuated that AI-driven solutions such as mental health applications and wearable devices allowed personalized treatment protocols, which could be generated according to real-time patient data integrations and patient-reported healthcare preferences. A patient dealing with anxiety, for example, could be prescribed tailored breathing techniques, mood-tracking feedback, and therapy suggestions powered by an AI that learns from their physiology and previous engagement history. This model adapts to patient needs to optimize treatment effectiveness and bolster engagement.

Developing digital psychiatry tools with the end-user in mind is crucial for usability and engagement. This includes:

- User-friendly interfaces that allow easy navigation through mental health apps.
- Emotion-aware AI that identifies feelings and reacts accordingly.
- Hybrid approach models designed to provide a balance between human guidance and AI free support services for mental healthcare.

A second crucial element of patient-centered digital psychiatry is autonomy and choice, controlling their mental health data, what type of interventions they will receive, and how much involvement AI will have in their care. If these principles are upheld, it fosters trust, adherence, and ongoing engagement with digital psychiatric solutions [74].

Ethics, equity, and patient-centered care are the foundational precepts of digital psychiatry upon which the responsible use of mental health technology rests. By framing the matching of mental models through rich contextual thinking, the chapter seeks to expedite a virtual play field, which can bridge the gap between accessibility and efficiency—the dichotomy that lies at the heart of all psychiatry, be it old or new. The continued growth in technology makes it imperative for us to maintain these principles so we can increase benefits and reduce risks for a more equitable, ethical, and patient-centered digital mental health marketplace.

7.5 Impacts of Digital Psychiatry on Mental Healthcare

Digital psychiatry is taking the rapid advance of enhancing accessibility, increasing engagement and acceptance of therapy, reducing the stigma of mental health, improving the personalized nature of human interaction and kicking into high gear. Digital psychiatry seeks to dismantle existing barriers in the delivery of mental healthcare using AI, mHealth applications, wearable technology, and telepsychiatry. We present herein an overview of important areas of transformation of the mental healthcare system and the patient experience by virtue of digital psychiatry.

7.5.1 Improving Accessibility and Affordability of Mental Health Services

Digital psychiatry works by filling gaps in our mental health landscape, particularly for people in rural, underserved, and low-resource settings [75]. Traditional psychiatric services are often plagued with issues such as long wait times, geographical limitations, and a scarcity of trained mental health professionals. Examples of telepsychiatry, AI-driven assessments, and mobile mental health apps are digital solutions that provide remote, on-demand care and access to mental health services to individuals, irrespective of their geographic locations [4], enhancing patient engagement and adherence to the treatment.

The cost of mental healthcare is another central obstacle that digital psychiatry is helping to overcome. Therapy sessions and psychiatric consultations in person are expensive, resulting in limited reach to a considerable portion of society especially for those not insured [76]. These AI-driven chatbots, mobile CBT apps, and self-guided digital interventions deliver cost-effective scalable automated support that can reach millions of users at once.

Additionally, government-backed telepsychiatry programs and employer-sponsored mental health platforms are integrating digital solutions to make psychiatric care more affordable and widely available [77]. As technology continues to evolve, the cost of AI-powered and digital interventions is expected to decrease, making high-quality mental healthcare more equitable and financially sustainable.

7.5.2 Reducing Stigma through Anonymous and Digital Interventions

Traditional psychiatric treatments often struggle with low adherence rates, as patients may discontinue medication or therapy due to lack of motivation, stigma, or logistical challenges. Digital psychiatry addresses this issue by providing personalized mental health interventions that engage users through AI-driven recommendations, real-time feedback, and gamified therapy experiences [78].

For instance, mHealth apps use daily reminders, mood-tracking features, and interactive CBT exercises to encourage patients to stay engaged with their treatment plans [79]. AI-driven mental health platforms analyze user behavior and adapt therapy sessions based on individual progress, ensuring a dynamic and patient-centric approach.

Wearable devices are becoming integrated into mental healthcare and also increase adherence passively capturing physiological and behavioral data. The data, collected by devices such as smartwatches, EEG headsets, and biosensors, get incorporated in real time, providing insight into metrics such as HRV, sleep, and physical activity—all of which can play a huge role in a patient's mental health. These data enable clinicians to use real-world physiological response to make changes to treatment plans for better patient outcomes and better patient compliance.

7.5.3 Personalized Medicine and Precision Psychiatry

Perhaps most encouraging of all, for the future of digital psychiatry, is the drive toward personalized medicine, whereby treatment is adjusted to individual differences in their psychological, biological, and environmental make-up. Predictive analytics and machine learning models driven by AI are changing psychiatric care by:

- Predicting mental health episodes before they occur using biometric and behavioral data
- Personalized medication plans derived from genetic and neurobiological profiles
- Improving therapy methods, driven by patient engagement as well as past treatment responses

AI algorithms, for example, are being created to pick up early warning signs of depression or psychosis by examining speech patterns, facial cues, and social media engagements [80]. This allows clinicians to take action earlier on, avoiding a deteriorating symptom presentation and better treatment results. Biometrics and digital phenotyping in psychiatry further the precision medicine approach [81]. For instance, the most common application of digital phenotyping is to analyze information regarding smartphone usage, movement patterns, voice tone, and typing speed to assess a person's mental health status [82]. Digital phenotyping allows for data-driven mental health interventions that are tailored to an individual's psychological state by continuously collecting objective, real-world data.

Although this transformation holds great promise, precision psychiatry stands to raise a number of ethical and privacy questions, and so its implementation must be supported by stringent data governance policies and robust regulatory oversight to develop equitable, transparent, and ethically sound procedures for informed consent [33].

7.5.4 Interdisciplinary Collaboration Between Psychiatry and Tech

The rapid growth of digital psychiatry has necessitated closer collaboration between mental health professionals, data scientists, software developers, and policymakers [20]. Interdisciplinary teams are essential to:

- Designing AI algorithms that are clinically validated and free from bias
- Developing user-friendly digital mental health applications that align with psychiatric principles
- Ensuring that technological innovations adhere to ethical, legal, and privacy standards

Medical institutions are increasingly incorporating digital psychiatry training for clinicians, ensuring that psychiatrists and therapists are equipped with the skills to interpret AI-driven insights, manage digital therapy platforms, and integrate technology into their practice [83].

The integration of technology in psychiatry also requires robust policies and legal frameworks to ensure safe, effective, and equitable implementation [84]. Governments and regulatory bodies must work alongside tech companies, mental health organizations, and medical professionals to establish:

- AI ethics guidelines for mental health applications
- Regulatory frameworks for DTx and telepsychiatry platforms
- Patient data protection policies that comply with global standards

By fostering strong public–private partnerships and cross-sector collaboration, digital psychiatry can continue to expand responsibly and equitably, ensuring long-term sustainability and societal impact [85].

The emergence of digital psychiatry has revolutionized mental healthcare by expanding access, increasing patient engagement, reducing stigma, allowing for personalized treatment, and encouraging interdisciplinary collaboration. Although the space offers huge potential, it will succeed only through ethical innovation, regulation, and further research. As psychiatry and technology continue to converge, an approach that is human-centric and inclusive will be critical to making sure that digital psychiatry is relevant and accessible to persons from all demographics and socioeconomic strata.

7.6 Applications and Use Cases

If you like something, please consider supporting me on Ko-Fi. These technologies facilitate early identification of mental health disorders, tailored interventions, and continual real-time monitoring of psychiatric conditions. Diagnostics, DTx platforms, and IoT-based monitoring systems are some of the branches that are applied in both clinical and real-world scenarios.

7.6.1 Diagnosis: Leveraging AI for Early Detection of Mental Health Disorders

Through extracting behaviors, language, and physiological patterns, AI is revolutionizing psychiatric diagnostics by detecting early signs of mental health disorders [86]. Standard psychiatric diagnosis is based largely on self-reporting of symptoms and observation by clinicians—methods that can be subjective and lagging. AI-powered models improve diagnostic accuracy by identifying subtle, objective signs of mental illness long before symptoms become acute.

Here are some potential uses of AI in psychiatric diagnosis:

- **NLP**: AI examines speech patterns, tone, linguistic markers to identify early signs of depression, schizophrenia, and cognitive decline For instance, changes in sentence structure, word choice, and speech fluency have been linked to mood disorders.
- **Facial and emotion recognition**: Machine learning algorithms assess microexpressions, eye movement, and facial muscle activity to identify emotional distress in patients. AI-driven tools such as Ellipsis Health and Affectiva are being explored for emotion recognition in mental health diagnostics.

- **Digital phenotyping**: Smartphones and wearables collect passive behavioral data, such as sleep patterns, physical activity, typing speed, and voice tone, to assess mental well-being. Studies show that changes in phone usage patterns and social media interactions can predict depressive episodes.

AI-powered diagnostic tools are being tested in clinical settings, workplaces, and telemedicine platforms. Hospitals and mental health clinics are integrating AI-based assessments into EHRs to assist psychiatrists in making data-driven diagnostic decisions [87].

However, challenges such as algorithmic bias, ethical concerns, and regulatory approvals must be addressed before AI-based diagnostics can be widely adopted. Ongoing research aims to validate these models across diverse populations to ensure fair and reliable mental health assessments.

7.6.2 Treatment: DTx and Virtual Care Platforms

DTx use software-based interventions to deliver evidence-based psychiatric treatments. These AI-powered platforms provide CBT, mindfulness exercises, and guided self-help interventions for conditions such as anxiety, depression, PTSD, and substance use disorders [88].

Notable AI-driven digital therapy solutions include:

- **Woebot**: An AI-powered chatbot that delivers conversational CBT through real-time, empathetic dialogue
- **Wysa**: A virtual mental health assistant that provides guided exercises for stress management, emotional regulation, and mindfulness
- **Ginger and Talkspace**: AI-assisted therapy platforms that connect patients with licensed therapists *via* text, voice, and video consultations

These solutions are particularly useful for individuals who cannot access traditional therapy due to cost, stigma, or geographical barriers.

7.6.3 Monitoring: Real-Time Patient Monitoring Using IoT Devices

IoT-enabled wearable devices and biosensors are revolutionizing mental health monitoring by collecting real-time physiological and behavioral data. These devices enable continuous, passive tracking of mental well-being, reducing the reliance on self-reported symptoms [89].

Common IoT-based mental health monitoring tools include:

- **Smartwatches (Apple Watch, Fitbit, Garmin)**: Measure HRV, sleep patterns, and physical activity to detect stress and mood fluctuations
- **EEG headbands (Muse, Emotiv)**: Analyze brainwave activity to assess anxiety levels and aid in relaxation training
- **Electrodermal activity sensors (Empatica E4, Biostrap)**: Monitor skin conductance responses, which are linked to emotional arousal and stress

These devices integrate with AI-powered analytics platforms that interpret biometric signals and provide personalized mental health recommendations.

Real-time patient monitoring using IoT devices is also being explored for suicide prevention and crisis intervention. AI algorithms analyze heart rate patterns, voice changes, and movement behavior to detect signs of acute distress. Some hospitals and research institutions are developing automated alert systems that notify caregivers or crisis response teams when high-risk individuals show warning signs of suicide or self-harm.

For example:

- Mindstrong Health is using smartphone data to detect cognitive and behavioral changes associated with depression and psychosis.
- BiAffect tracks smartphone keyboard dynamics to identify mood changes in individuals with bipolar disorder.

Although IoT devices provide valuable insights into mental health, challenges such as data privacy, false positives, and user compliance must be addressed. Continuous monitoring raises ethical concerns about surveillance and consent, requiring transparent data-sharing policies and regulatory oversight.

Moreover, integration with clinical workflows remains a challenge, as many psychiatric care providers lack the infrastructure to process large volumes of wearable-generated data. Future research must focus on standardizing IoT data interpretation and integrating it into mainstream psychiatric care.

The use of AI, DTx, and IoT in digital psychiatry is revolutionizing the way mental health disorders are diagnosed, treated, and monitored. AI-driven early detection models improve diagnostic accuracy, digital therapy platforms make mental healthcare more scalable and accessible, and IoT-based wearables enable continuous, real-time tracking of psychiatric conditions.

However, challenges such as ethical concerns, data security, clinical validation, and regulatory compliance must be addressed to ensure the responsible and equitable deployment of these technologies. Moving forward, interdisciplinary collaboration between psychiatrists, AI researchers, and regulatory bodies will be key to maximizing the benefits and minimizing the risks of digital psychiatry.

7.6.4 Prevention: Technology-Driven Risk Assessment and Preventive Strategies

Preventive psychiatry focuses on identifying and mitigating mental health risks before they develop into severe disorders. Emerging AI-driven risk assessment models, digital screening tools, and IoT-based early warning systems are revolutionizing prevention strategies by enabling real-time mental health tracking, early intervention, and personalized wellness plans. These technologies help identify at-risk individuals, predict mental health crises, and implement preventive measures at both individual and population levels [90].

AI and machine learning are being increasingly utilized to analyze behavioral, social, and physiological data to predict mental health risks. By examining historical patient records, digital phenotyping data, and real-time biometric indicators, AI models can identify patterns associated with depression, anxiety, PTSD, and suicide risk.

Some key AI-driven prevention methods are:

- **Speech and text analysis**: NLP algorithms powered by AI analyze speech patterns, social media activity, and text messages to identify indications of emotional distress or suicidal thoughts. Linguistic markers, including negative sentiment, slowed speech, and heightened self-referential language, have been found to predict depressive episodes.
- **Social media and digital behavior monitoring**: Studies have shown that social media activity, late-night phone behavior, and search history trends can all be potential indicators of poor mental health. Based on this information, AI algorithms examine these digital behaviors to direct tailored enhancements to emotional well-being or guides for emergency scenarios.
- **Machine learning–based suicide prediction models**: AI models, derived using EHRs, demographic details, and psychiatric history, have shown high accuracy in predicting individuals vulnerable to suicidal behavior.

These models assist clinicians in performing early management of high-risk patients.

Although these tools show great promise, significant ethical issues including privacy, bias in AI predictions, and consent in digital surveillance must be carefully handled. Ensuring that AI-based insights are acting ethically and efficiently will always require human oversight.

One area of healthcare that is seeing a huge transformation is preventive mental healthcare, where wearable devices and IoT systems have enabled continuous monitoring of physiological and behavioral signals that indicate early symptoms of stress, anxiety, and depression. The solution provides real-time monitoring of these high-risk patients, providing for data-driven preventive interventions reducing the chance of significant psychiatric episodes.

Preventive strategies based on IoT include the following key principles:

- **HRV and stress detection**: Smartwatches and biosensors follow HRV, skin conductance, and corticosterone levels—generic biomarkers of chronic stress and anxiety conditions. Wellness AI analytics help users detect what triggers stress and achieve coping habits before symptoms get worse.
- **Sleep and mood monitoring**: Changes in the pattern of sleep are good predictors of mental health disorders (eg, bipolar disorder, depression, schizophrenia) Wearables such as Fitbit, Oura Ring, and Apple Watch track sleep cycles and offer tailored guidance on enhancing mental fitness.
- **Voice and facial recognition for emotional monitoring**: Some emerging technologies utilize AI to analyze the face and voice tone detect whether there is any change in the mood of a patient. These systems notify users or clinicians when early signs of distress

are identified, which allows for preventive intervention before a crisis occurs.

Although IoT-based solutions provide the advantage of early intervention, issues of continuous surveillance, data privacy, and agency should be managed *via* transparent user consent and secure data archiving process.

In addition to risk assessment, digital psychiatry is fostering proactive mental health interventions through AI-driven self-help tools, digital mental wellness programs, and gamified behavioral therapies.

Some key preventive interventions include:

- **Personalized mental wellness apps**: AI-driven apps such as Youper, Mindstrong, and Woebot use adaptive learning algorithms to provide personalized mental health coaching, early symptom tracking, and preventive therapy exercises. These tools empower users to develop resilience and manage stress before symptoms worsen.
- **Mindfulness and digital CBT platforms**: Apps such as Headspace, Calm, and Moodfit integrate AI-driven insights to offer tailored meditation, breathing exercises, and CBT modules that help users prevent anxiety and depressive episodes.
- **Workplace mental health and burnout prevention**: Companies are increasingly integrating digital wellness platforms that use AI to monitor employee stress levels, detect burnout risk, and suggest preventive well-being strategies such as break reminders, relaxation techniques, and workload management tools.

These digital interventions empower individuals to take control of their mental health, shifting psychiatric care from a reactive to a proactive model.

Beyond individual interventions, technology is playing a pivotal role in population-level mental health prevention through big data analytics, AI-driven mental health surveillance, and digital public health campaigns.

Key initiatives include:

- **Predictive mental health analytics for policy making**: Governments and public health agencies use AI to analyze mental health trends across regions and allocate resources where psychiatric care is most needed.
- **Crisis helplines and AI-based suicide prevention programs**: Organizations such as Crisis Text Line and Samaritans are leveraging AI algorithms to analyze direct chat data from helpline users and identify high-risk individuals to offer immediate support.
- **AI in school and university mental health programs**: AI-powered platforms for student well-being allow colleges and universities to identify early symptoms of anxiety, stress, or depression and provide preventive services to at-risk students.

When matched with AI-powered actionable insight data at scale, public health organizations can create more effective mental health prevention programs and help reduce the financial burden of psychiatric disorders worldwide. As technology-driven prevention strategies are revolutionizing mental healthcare, they also pose a number of challenges:

- **Privacy and data security**: Monitoring mental health data comes with ethical implications around surveillance, consent, and data misuse, by ensuring patient privacy and securing data under regulatory frameworks such as HIPAA and GDPR.
- **Algorithmic bias and fairness**: Risk assessment AI models must not only be trained but also trained on diverse, representative datasets to prevent biased prediction and skewed decision trees affecting vulnerable populations.

- **Integration with traditional psychiatric care**: Digital preventive strategies should complement—not supplant—human-centered psychiatric interventions, thus ensuring that technology augments clinical decision-making rather than replaces professional judgment.
- **Long-term efficacy and validation**: Many AI-driven preventive tools require longitudinal studies to assess their long-term effectiveness, accuracy, and impact on psychiatric outcomes.

As digital psychiatry continues to evolve, addressing these challenges will be critical in ensuring that technology-driven prevention strategies are ethical, effective, and widely accessible.

Technology-driven risk assessment and prevention are revolutionizing mental healthcare by shifting the focus from reactive treatment to proactive intervention. AI-powered diagnostic models, IoT-based monitoring tools, and DTx interventions provide real-time insights, personalized mental wellness plans, and large-scale public health solutions.

However, to fully realize the potential of preventive digital psychiatry, a multistakeholder approach involving clinicians, AI researchers, policymakers, and ethicists is necessary. By ensuring privacy, fairness, and seamless integration with traditional psychiatric care, these technologies can reduce the global burden of mental health disorders and improve long-term well-being.

7.7 Benefits and Opportunities

The integration of AI, mHealth, wearable technology, and big data analytics into psychiatry has revolutionized mental healthcare. Digital psychiatry offers enhanced access, cost-effective scalability, data-driven personalization, and continuous innovation, enabling a more inclusive, efficient, and patient-centered approach to mental healthcare. This section explores the key benefits and future opportunities that digital psychiatry presents.

7.7.1 Enhanced Access to Care

Traditional psychiatric care faces significant challenges related to limited availability of mental health professionals, long wait times, and geographical barriers. Digital psychiatry addresses these issues by providing remote, AI-driven, and automated interventions, ensuring that individuals can receive support regardless of their location or socioeconomic status.

Key ways digital psychiatry enhances accessibility include:

- **Telepsychiatry and online therapy platforms**: Services such as Talkspace, BetterHelp, and Ginger enable patients to connect with licensed therapists remotely, making psychiatric support more accessible [91].
- **AI-powered mental health chatbots**: AI-driven platforms such as Woebot and Wysa provide 24/7 mental health support, offering evidence-based interventions at scale [92].
- **mHealth apps for self-guided therapy**: Digital CBT, mindfulness apps, and emotional wellness trackers provide low-cost, on-demand mental health resources for users who may not seek traditional therapy [79].

By expanding the reach of mental healthcare beyond clinical settings, digital psychiatry reduces disparities and ensures mental health support is available to more people globally.

Another advantage of digital psychiatry is its potential to provide culturally relevant, multilingual mental health interventions [93]. Many AI-driven therapy platforms now incorporate language translation, cultural adaptation, and region-specific therapeutic models to cater to diverse populations. This ensures that individuals from different ethnic, linguistic, and socioeconomic backgrounds receive personalized and contextually appropriate mental health support.

7.7.2 Scalability and Cost-Effectiveness

Mental health treatment is often expensive and inaccessible, particularly in low-income and uninsured populations [83]. Digital psychiatry significantly reduces the cost of psychiatric interventions by leveraging AI-driven automation, virtual care platforms, and scalable mobile applications.

Key cost-saving advantages include:

- **Lower therapy costs**: AI-driven therapy chatbots and DTx provide affordable alternatives to traditional therapy [83].
- **Reduced need for in-person consultations**: Telepsychiatry and digital mental health platforms minimize hospital visits, travel expenses, and associated costs [94].
- **Early detection and preventive interventions**: AI-powered risk assessment models and wearable monitoring devices enable early intervention, reducing the long-term costs associated with untreated psychiatric conditions [29].

By leveraging technology-driven automation, digital psychiatry allows governments, healthcare systems, and employers to provide mental health support at scale without incurring high costs.

One of the most significant opportunities in digital psychiatry is its ability to scale mental health services efficiently [95]. Unlike traditional therapy, which is time-intensive and limited by clinician availability, digital platforms serve thousands of users simultaneously with minimal human intervention.

Examples of scalable digital psychiatric interventions include:

- **AI-based mental health screening in workplaces and schools**: AI-driven mental health assessments enable large-scale mental health screenings to detect at-risk individuals early [96].

- **Digital public health campaigns and crisis response systems**: Governments and nongovernmental organizations are using AI-powered mental health hotlines and crisis intervention chatbots to provide instant mental health support at scale [97].
- **Remote psychiatric services for disaster and conflict zones**: Digital psychiatry solutions enable mental health support in war zones, refugee camps, and areas affected by natural disasters, where traditional services may be unavailable [98].

Scalability ensures that mental health interventions reach broader populations, significantly improving global mental health outcomes.

7.7.3 Data-Driven Personalization of Treatments

The shift toward precision psychiatry enables treatments to be tailored to an individual's genetic, behavioral, and neurophysiological profiles [99]. Machine learning models analyze biometric data, mood patterns, and therapy engagement to recommend personalized interventions that improve treatment efficacy.

Key advances in data-driven personalization include:

- **AI-based treatment matching**: Algorithms analyze clinical history and symptom patterns to recommend the treatment approach, whether CBT, medication, or behavioral therapy [100].
- **Wearable-driven mood tracking and adaptive interventions**: Real-time biometric and behavioral data from wearables help adjust treatment plans based on sleep patterns, HRV, and stress levels [101].
- **Genetic and neuroimaging-based precision psychiatry**: AI-powered analysis of genetic markers and neuroimaging scans is helping to predict medication responses and optimize psychiatric treatment plans [29].

AI-driven feedback loops allow mental health interventions to adapt dynamically based on user interactions [102]. This ensures that digital therapy sessions, mindfulness exercises, and cognitive interventions evolve to match an individual's progress and mental health state.

For example:

- mHealth apps adjust therapy modules based on mood tracking data and therapy completion rates [103].
- AI-powered chatbots modify conversation styles based on user sentiment analysis and engagement patterns [104].
- Wearable-based interventions suggest breathing exercises or meditation when stress levels rise [105].

Personalized treatments enhance patient engagement, adherence, and overall effectiveness, improving long-term mental health outcomes.

7.7.4 Opportunities for Continuous Innovation

The future of digital psychiatry will be driven by more advanced AI models capable of understanding and responding to complex emotional states. Future NLP models will enable:

- **Emotionally intelligent AI therapists**: AI chatbots with advanced emotion recognition and deep psychological understanding [106]
- **Automated real-time sentiment analysis**: AI-driven text, voice, and facial analysis to detect and intervene in moments of crisis [107]
- **Multimodal AI for holistic mental health assessment**: Combining text, voice, facial expression, and biometric data for enhanced psychiatric evaluations [108]

Upcoming innovations in mental health wearables and neurotechnology will enhance psychiatric care by:

- **BCIs for mood regulation**: Emerging BCIs offer potential noninvasive neuromodulation for treating depression, PTSD, and anxiety [109]
- **Smart textiles and biometric sensors**: Wearable fabrics embedded with biometric sensors to track stress levels, cortisol release, and physiological responses [110]
- **Neural and digital biomarker discovery**: AI-driven brain imaging and neurophysiological signal processing for early mental disorder detection [111]

The continuous development of ethical AI frameworks, regulatory policies, and patient-centric digital interventions will ensure that digital psychiatry evolves responsibly and equitably. Key focus areas include:

- **Bias reduction in AI models**: Ensuring fair, unbiased, and diverse AI datasets
- **Privacy-preserving AI techniques**: Using federated learning and blockchain to enhance data security and patient confidentiality
- **Human-centered AI regulation**: Establishing international ethical guidelines for AI-driven mental health interventions

The combination of new technologies, the findings of modern neuroscience, conclusively indicates that psychiatry is on the verge of a very substantial transformation, which will inevitably open new doors for mental healthcare. Although challenges associated with data privacy, AI bias, and clinical validation still persist, continuous research and interdisciplinary collaboration will secure that digital psychiatry will be ethical, effective, and broadly available.

7.8 Challenges and Limitations

Although digital psychiatry has made tremendous progress, there are still many challenges and limitations that make it hard to adopt or be effective. Thoughtful attention regarding ethics, implementation, regulation, acceptability, and accessibility is needed to enable opportunities for safe and equitable digital psychiatry. This section analyzes some of the core challenges and their impact on digital mental healthcare going forward. Table 7.3 highlights the advantages and potential drawbacks of digital psychiatry across key dimensions.

7.8.1 Ethical Dilemmas: Data Privacy and Algorithmic Bias

Data privacy and security constitute one of the most pressing ethical issues in digital psychiatry. Platforms for digital mental health, AI assessments, and wearable technologies gather sensitive psychological, physiological, and behavioral data [35]. These data can be misused, leaked, or exploited by third parties if not properly handled, increasing concerns that include the following:

Table 7.3 Contrasting the strengths and shortcomings of digital psychiatry adoption.

Category	Benefits	Limitations
Accessibility	Reaches remote and underserved areas	Dependent on digital literacy
Affordability	Reduces long-term care costs	Requires initial tech investment
Personalization	AI-driven, adaptive therapy	Risk of overreliance on algorithms
Data-driven insights	Real-time monitoring and feedback	Privacy concerns
Scalability	Can support large populations efficiently	Requires strong infrastructure

- Cyberattacks are also targeting mental health databases.
- A lack of transparency in AI decision-making leads to possible attacks on patient data.
- Poorly designed consent processes: Users may not understand how their data are used.

To mitigate these risks, it is essential to implement:

- Secure data storage and transmission with end-to-end encryption
- Federated learning to train AI models using decentralized patient data, without exposing raw data
- To heavily abide by privacy laws (HIPAA, GDPR) to govern data collection and sharing

Due to limited datasets used in digital psychiatry, AI models used in the detection of mental disorders may not represent specific populations, which can lead to algorithmic bias with regard to detecting mental disorders. Biased models can result in:

- Misdiagnoses or inaccurate predictions, especially among groups that are racially, gender or socioeconomically diverse
- Heavy reliance on western-dominated data, making it less effective in non-western cultures
- AI-based mental health recommendations that do not adjust for variances in how people experience symptoms

To improve fairness and equity, AI models must:

- Have been trained under diverse, global representative datasets
- Subject to ongoing auditing and bias detection by an interdisciplinary team of experts

- Embrace explainability tools that facilitate understanding of AI-driven decisions by clinicians and patients

If not addressed, ethical concerns related to privacy breaches and biased AI models may reduce trust in digital psychiatry, limiting its adoption and effectiveness.

7.8.2 Technological Challenges: Integration, Interoperability, and Infrastructure

Although AI and digital tools hold great promise, incorporating these technologies into the existing psychiatric workflow is challenging. Mental health providers do not have the infrastructure, technical know-how, or standardized frameworks to integrate seamlessly:

- AI-powered diagnostics into clinical practice
- Incorporation of IoT-based patient monitoring systems in psychiatric treatment plans
- Interoperable EHRs linking digital psychiatry tools with hospitals and clinics

When it comes to improving adoption, healthcare systems need to:

- Establish uniform protocols for the integration of digital psychiatry
- Provide mental health professionals with AI and DTx literacy
- Enable seamless integrations between digital psychiatry platforms and hospital EHRs

Several low-resource places do not have the technology infrastructure necessary for digital psychiatry (for this to proceed, the following need to be present):

- Stable internet connectivity for telepsychiatry and mHealth apps
- High-processing power data centers for AI-driven mental health analytics
- Appropriate cybersecurity safeguards to protect sensitive psychiatric information

This is a divide where public–private partnerships can help with investments in digital mental health systems and cost-effective and scalable solutions for resource-limited settings.

7.8.3 Regulatory and Legal Hurdles

Regulatory schemas for AI-based mental health diagnosis, DTx, and telepsychiatry vary greatly across different nations. Current challenges include:

- Coherence around AI liability in psychiatric misdiagnoses
- Diverse telemedicine laws impeding the global growth of digital psychiatry platforms
- No established approval pathways for AI enhanced mental health solutions. Governments and regulatory agencies need to:
    - Define a legal framework for digital psychiatry and AI-based mental health solutions
    - Establish agreements for global data sharing while respecting robust privacy protections
    - Develop AI accountability and liability frameworks to protect the patient

In the absence of strong regulation, there is a risk of widespread use of unvalidated AI models and unethical digital mental health practices compromising patient outcome.

7.8.4 Resistance to Adoption Among Patients and Practitioners

Many mental health practitioners are reluctant to adopt AI psych tools for reasons such as:

- Fear of losing jobs, with AI taking over functions of human therapists
- Trust in AI-driven diagnoses and treatment recommendations
- Concerns about diminished human contact in online mental health interventions

To counter such resistance, digital psychiatry needs to be framed as a supplement, not a substitute for patient-centered care. Solutions include:

- Emphasizing AI-human hybrids rather than AI that replaces psychiatric decision-making
- Training programs to assist clinicians in interpreting AI-driven insights
- Designing ethical AI, by making sure that human empathy will continue at the heart of digital mental healthcare

As a result, many patients are skeptical about AI-powered therapy chatbots, remote mental health monitoring capabilities, and DTx because of the following:

- Concerns over the potential misuse of data and fear of privacy infringement
- Trusting AI and using it for therapy interventions
- Minimal digital skills, particularly among elderly people or disadvantaged groups

For adoption, digital psychiatry platforms must:

- Increase transparency around how AI-based interventions operate
- Introduce convenient mental health applications with easy-to-use interfaces
- Raise awareness among patients about the merits and safety protocols surrounding digital mental health resources

However, overcoming these obstacles will be critical for establishing trust and engagement in digital psychiatric solutions.

7.8.5 Digital Divide: Bridging Gaps in Accessibility

Despite these advancements, access to digital psychiatric tools remains limited for many people—especially in rural areas, in low-income communities, and in developing countries—because of:

- Not having a smartphone, internet, or the technology in their home
- Development needs of AI-based mental health apps and wearables
- Language and cultural challenges in digital mental health platforms. To ensure digital psychiatry is inclusive, it must be:
    - Create zero-rate, offline-functioning apps for the mental well-being of communities with limited internet access.
    - Provide low cost or free mental health apps to low-income populations.

Provide multilingual AI therapy models that take into consideration how culture defines psychiatric care.

Instead, they may deepen mental health disparities by depriving vulnerable populations of critical psychiatric support. Despite the promise of digital psychiatry, there are important ethical, technical, legal, and accessibility challenges to be met such that digital psychiatry is responsibly, equitably, and effectively implemented. To push through these limitations, need to:

- Stronger regulation in AI and digital mental health interventions
- Development of ethical AI for fairness, privacy, and transparency
- Infrastructure investments to widen digital psychiatric services to underserved populations
- Interdisciplinary collaboration among psychiatrists, AI researchers, policymakers, and technologists is essential to ensure that digital psychiatry solutions are clinically relevant, ethically sound, and technically robust.

Digital psychiatry has the potential to improve mental health globally if it addresses these challenges and limitations and retains technology as a tool and not a replacement for human-based psychiatric care.

7.9 Future Directions

The combination of generative AI with existing mental health support systems is one of the most promising use cases of digital psychiatry. Unlike conventional AI chatbots, generative AI models such as ChatGPT, Bard, and AI-powered therapy assistants are maturing to deliver contextual, emotionally intelligent responses. They will also empower users in a meaningful conversation and tailor responses based on real-time sentiment analysis and user history. With multiple patient interactions, future AI therapy models could learn and augment their approach to offer tailor-made interventions by a compassionate monitor.

An emerging frontier in psychiatry is the advent of BCIs. BCIs provide a direct means of communication between the brain and external devices, allowing for real-time feedback and intervention for psychiatric disorders. Corporate players such as Neuralink and Kernel are creating user-friendly BCIs that gather noninvasive data about neural activity correlated with mood disorders, PTSD, and schizophrenia. In the next decade, BCIs may enable people to control their emotional states, providing a nonpharmaceutical option to mental healthcare. Such developments could be extremely beneficial for patients with treatment-resistant depression and anxiety disorders.

Digital psychiatry could overcome mental health inequities and provide psychiatric services to underserved populations globally. And millions are without adequate care, as large parts of the world have a serious shortage of mental health professionals. The technology is highly promising, and the need for AI-based digital psychiatry solutions to scale the provision of psychiatric support in low-resource settings is becoming increasingly urgent—be it in the form of automatic screening tools, remote telepsychiatry services, or mental health assessments deployed on cyberspace platforms. Long-term innovation will be in the area of developing cheap, multilingual, and culturally responsive AI models that will cater to a diverse global populace.

A further important impact area will be the integration of digital psychiatry in public health. AI-based systems that surveil the mental health of populations are increasingly being adopted by governments and global health organizations to detect trends in emerging mental illness and suicide risk. By examining large-scale datasets—from social media activity to interactions with crisis hotlines to behavioral health records—these systems can predict and prevent large-scale mental health crises. Such action could help curb suicide, substance use, and psychiatric hospitalization on a global level.

The case for quantum computing in mental diagnosis thus first requires a nod to the massive amounts of data that can be captured and analyzed in seconds, far outpacing traditional methods of data analysis. The characterization of psychiatric disorders such as schizophrenia, bipolar disorder, or major depressive disorder is a problem of multiple causations and requires sorting through large collections of data such as genetic data, neuroimaging scans, and behavioral markers. Quantum computing will enable researchers to analyze these vast multidimensional datasets in real time, revealing hidden patterns in psychiatric disorders.

One of the most anticipated breakthroughs from quantum-powered AI models is their ability to predict psychiatric disorders with unprecedented accuracy. At present, AI models that form the backbone of diagnosis are linear computations that are not well suited to identify the intricacies of genetic, environmental, and behavioral risk factors that increase the odds for mental illnesses. Quantum computing will enable more accurate assessments of individual psychiatric risk tailored to the specific profile of the patient, and will suggest a probable course of treatment and when to implement it. Finally, quantum computing can expedite the discovery of psychiatric medications, allowing pharmaceutical companies to create more effective treatments for mental disorders by modeling neurochemical interactions at a molecular level.

Despite its potential, quantum computing in psychiatry remains in its infancy, with significant challenges in practical implementation, cost, and accessibility. However, as the technology matures, it is expected to play a pivotal role in transforming mental health research and clinical applications.

The COVID-19 pandemic has highlighted an urgent need for mental health solutions that can deliver routine care at times of crisis. Lockdowns, economic instability, and social isolation triggered a worldwide mental health crisis that laid bare deficits in conventional models of psychiatric care. Telepsychiatry, AI-enabled crisis hotlines and digital therapy platforms, in turn, became essential lifelines for millions of people experiencing anxiety, depression, and trauma. Kaiser, M.D., M.P.H., Senior Psychiatric Consultant, VA National Center for PTSD. Disaster and Crisis Response: Digital Psychiatry. Moving forward, we anticipate that digital psychiatry will play an increasingly important role in disaster and crisis response efforts.

A significant breakthrough in this domain is the creation of AI-assisted psychological resilience training solutions. These initiatives use machine learning and behavioral insights to assist individuals in developing coping mechanisms ahead of crises. AI-driven mental health coaching can offer tailored stress management strategies, mindfulness practices, and adaptable coping mechanisms to mitigate psychological distress in future pandemics or disasters. Similarly, wearable technology can be deployed to assess frontline workers' stress levels, enabling organizations to intervene early and preventing burnout and PTSD.

One of the most groundbreaking developments in this area is the development of AI bots that can help train individuals to be psychologically resilient. These initiatives use machine learning and behavioral insights to help people build coping skills before crises. Tailored stress management strategies, mindfulness practices, and adaptive coping mechanisms can be integrated to reduce psychiatric distress in future pandemics and disasters by using AI-powered mental health coaching. Analogous to this, wearables can also help to monitor stress levels of frontline workers so that organizations can proactively intervene and prevent burnout and PTSD.

Since there have been enormous changes to the future of digital psychiatry, from generative AI-driven therapy models to BCIs and quantum-powered psychiatric research, new technology promises to transform the diagnosis, treatment, and prevention of mental health disorders. The international proliferation of virtual mental health services will help alleviate access disparities and improve mental healthcare internationally.

These advancements alone are not a guarantee of progress and must be accompanied by principles of compassionate and unbiased implementation, including duly vigilant regulation and oversight, as well as grassroots-level equitable distribution. Ensuring that AI models are free of bias, that quantum computing is put to use responsibly, and that tools to determine the steps toward response to crisis are universally available will be critical in maximizing the benefits of digital psychiatry. Future digital psychiatry should embrace interprofessional team-based approach and innovative technology-driven approach.

7.10 Conclusion

Digital psychiatry refers to a shift in the paradigm of mental healthcare, leveraging AI, wearable technology, digital therapeutics, and computational models to advance the diagnosis, treatment, and prevention of psychiatric disorders. In this chapter, we have reviewed the foundations, technological advances, applications, benefits, and challenges of digital psychiatry, thus offering insight into its transformative impact on the mental health landscape. With the advancement of technology, its incorporation in psychiatry has the incredible potential to transform the delivery of mental health services, rendering them more accessible, personalized, and data-driven.

More data can lead to more subtle signals, such as AI and machine learning to improve early detection, keep real-time tabs on the patient, and customize treatment plans. Digital psychiatry has already shown enormous promise in telepsychiatry, AI-assisted diagnostics, mobile mental health apps, and VR therapy. If anything, new technologies such as BCIs, quantum computing, or generative AI will only improve the accuracy, efficiency, and scalability of this emerging form of psychiatric care. Nevertheless, ethical concerns, data security issues, legal challenges, and digital inequity continue to be significant barriers that need to be addressed to facilitate the responsible and equitable use of these technologies.

Nonetheless, the transformative power of technology in psychiatry is profound. AI-enabled chatbots are offering round-the-clock mental health support, wearables biosensors are facilitating continuous reporting of psychiatric symptoms diagnostics, and blockchain is improving data privacy and protection. Finally, quantum computing, combined with neurotechnology, could result in extended mental health research, high-precision diagnostics, and novel therapy mechanisms. If used responsibly, these breakthroughs can democratize mental healthcare, particularly for some of the most at-risk groups in society.

Looking ahead, it is important to notice that the various stakeholders need to collaborate to ensure that we maximize the benefits of digital psychiatry, while minimizing its risks. Clinicians should adopt digital tools as an addition to traditional psychiatry but maintain that human oversight is the core of mental healthcare. They should create ethical AIs, minimizing biases and, at the same time, elaborating the transparency of digital interventions. We have a responsibility as policymakers to create strong regulations and global standards on the practice of the electronic and mobile psychiatry established around the world so that mental health technologies are safe, effective, and inclusive to the public. With collaboration, these stakeholders can pave the way for better and universal mental healthcare that is innovative and responsive to local issues.

The future of psychiatry will be a balance between human experience and technological advancement. Digital psychiatry can address existing gaps in mental healthcare delivery by embracing ethical, patient-centered innovation, thereby enabling a more inclusive, scalable, and effective mental health ecosystem. This was only the first step toward a positive psychiatric revolution with the help of tech—it is time for stakeholders to take action, be creative, and maintain the establishment of the future of mental healthcare to not only be revolutionary, but human-centric as well.

AI disclosure statement: The author acknowledges the use of AI-based tools for minor language editing or grammatical correction. However, all intellectual contributions, analyses, and conclusions presented in this chapter are entirely the author's own.

Bibliography

1. Philippe, T.J., Sikder, N., Jackson, A., Koblanski, M.E., Liow, E., Pilarinos, A., Vasarhelyi, K., Digital health interventions for delivery of mental health care: Systematic and comprehensive meta-review. *JMIR Ment. Health*, 9, 5, e35159, 2022.
2. Onnela, J.-P. and Rauch, S.L., Harnessing smartphone-based digital phenotyping to enhance behavioral and mental health. *Neuropsychopharmacology*, 41, 7, 1691–1696, 2016.

3. Burr, C., Taddeo, M., Floridi, L., The ethics of digital well-being: A thematic review. *Sci. Eng. Ethics*, 26, 4, 2313–2343, 2020.
4. Pavlopoulos, A., Rachiotis, T., Maglogiannis, I., An overview of tools and technologies for anxiety and depression management using AI. *Appl. Sci.*, 14, 19, 9068, 2024.
5. Muhammad, F. and Arafat, S.Y., Technology-based interventions for mental health support in bangladesh, in: *Mental health in Bangladesh: From bench to community*, pp. 271–291, Springer, Cham, Switzerland, 2024.
6. Chivilgina, O., Elger, B.S., Jotterand, F., Digital technologies for schizophrenia management: A descriptive review. *Sci. Eng. Ethics*, 27, 1–22, 2021.
7. Oyeniyi, J. and Oluwaseyi, P., Emerging trends in ai-powered medical imaging: enhancing diagnostic accuracy and treatment decisions. *Int. J. Enhanced Res. Sci. Technol. Eng.*, 13, 2319–7463, 2024.
8. Fischer, A., Data sovereignty and e-governance: The legal implications of national laws on digital government systems. *Legal Stud. Digital Age*, 2, 4, 1–12, 2023.
9. Wainberg, M.L., Scorza, P., Shultz, J.M., Helpman, L., Mootz, J.J., Johnson, K.A., Neria, Y., Bradford, J.-M.E., Oquendo, M.A., Arbuckle, M.R., Challenges and opportunities in global mental health: A research-to-practice perspective. *Curr. Psychiatry Rep.*, 19, 1–10, 2017.
10. Balcombe, L. and De Leo, D., Digital mental health challenges and the horizon ahead for solutions. *JMIR Mental Health*, 8, 3, e26811, 2021.
11. Ahmed, Z., Telepsychiatry: A new frontier in mental health care delivery and access. *Front. Healthcare Technol.*, 1, 01, 1–12, 2024.
12. Zulkarnain, R., Hardi, R., Syabandyah, F., Rahayu, H., Herawati, H., *et al.*, AI-powered smart smile: Early detection of mental health conditions through computational intelligence, in: *2024 18th International Conference on Telecommunication Systems, Services, and Applications (TSSA)*, IEEE, pp. 1–6, 2024.
13. Olawade, D.B., Wada, O.Z., Odetayo, A., David-Olawade, A.C., Asaolu, F., Eberhardt, J., Enhancing mental health with artificial intelligence: Current trends and future prospects. *J. Med. Surg. Public Health*, 100099, 2024.
14. Patibandla, R.L., Bhuyan, H.K., Rao, B.T., Murthy, M.R., Proactive prognosis: Predicting the course of mental and neurological disorders with artificial intelligence, in: *Revolutionizing Medical Systems using*

Artificial Intelligence, pp. 75–92, Elsevier, Amsterdam, Netherlands, 2025.

15. Jafleh, E.A., Alnaqbi, F.A., Almaeeni, H.A., Faqeeh, S., Alzaabi, M.A., Al Zaman, K., Alnaqbi, F., Almaeeni, H., Alzaabi, M., The role of wearable devices in chronic disease monitoring and patient care: A comprehensive review. *Cureus*, 16, 9, 2024.
16. Mitsea, E., Drigas, A., Skianis, C., Digitally assisted mindfulness in training self-regulation skills for sustainable mental health: A systematic review. *Behav. Sci.*, 13, 12, 1008, 2023.
17. Singha, R. and Singha, S., Mental health treatment: Exploring the potential of augmented reality and virtual reality, in: *Applications of Virtual and Augmented Reality for Health and Wellbeing*, pp. 91–110, IGI Global, Hershey, Pennsylvania, USA, 2024.
18. Li, W., Yigitcanlar, T., Browne, W., Nili, A., The making of responsible innovation and technology: An overview and framework. *Smart Cities*, 6, 4, 1996–2034, 2023.
19. Almira, O.T., Evaluating virtual reality and artificial intelligence as emerging digital tools for mental health care, 2025.
20. Stein, D.J., Shoptaw, S.J., Vigo, D.V., Lund, C., Cuijpers, P., Bantjes, J., Sartorius, N., Maj, M., Psychiatric diagnosis and treatment in the 21st century: Paradigm shifts versus incremental integration. *World Psychiatry*, 21, 3, 393–414, 2022.
21. Burley, J., Hughes, J.J., Stubbs, A., Eisikovits, N., The ethics of automating therapy, 2024.
22. Andersson, G., Internet interventions: past, present and future. *Internet Interventions*, 12, 181–188, 2018.
23. Mucic, D., Hilty, D.M., Parish, M.B., Yellowlees, P.M., Web-and internet-based services: Education, support, self care, and formal treatment approaches. *e-Mental Health*, 173–192, 2016.
24. Karimian, M., *et al.*, A short review on diagnosing and predicting mental disorders with machine learning. *Int. J. Appl. Data Sci. Eng. Health*, 1, 1, 20–27, 2025.
25. Sheikh, M., Qassem, M., Kyriacou, P.A., Wearable, environmental, and smartphone-based passive sensing for mental health monitoring. *Front. Digital Health*, 3, 662811, 2021.
26. Liu, Y., Liu, R., Ge, J., Wang, Y., Advancements in brain-machine interfaces for application in the metaverse. *Front. Neurosci.*, 18, 1383319, 2024.

27. Fusar-Poli, P., Manchia, M., Koutsouleris, N., Leslie, D., Woopen, C., Calkins, M.E., Dunn, M., Le Tourneau, C., Mannikko, M., Mollema, T., *et al.*, Ethical considerations for precision psychiatry: A roadmap for research and clinical practice. *Eur. Neuropsychopharmacol.*, 63, 17–34, 2022.
28. Wong, A., Chan, I., Tsang, C.H., Chan, A.Y., Shum, A.K., Lai, E.S., Yip, P., A local review on the use of a bio-psycho-social model in school-based mental health promotion. *Front. Psychiatry*, 12, 691815, 2021.
29. Omiyefa, S., Artificial intelligence and machine learning in precision mental health diagnostics and predictive treatment models. *Int. J. Res. Publ. Rev.*, 6, 3, 85–99, 2025.
30. Zeine, F. and Changizi, S., Awareness integration theory meets AI-driven technology for advanced mental health solutions. *Technol. Educ.*, 106, 2024.
31. Mirabdolah, A., Alaeifard, M., Marandi, A., User-centered design in hcl: Enhancing usability and interaction in complex systems. *Int. J. Adv. Hum. Comput. Interact.*, 1, 1, 16–33, 2023.
32. Bufano, P., Laurino, M., Said, S., Tognetti, A., Menicucci, D., Digital phenotyping for monitoring mental disorders: Systematic review. *J. Med. Internet Res.*, 25, e46778, 2023.
33. Galderisi, S., Appelbaum, P.S., Gill, N., Gooding, P., Herrman, H., Melillo, A., Myrick, K., Pathare, S., Savage, M., Szmukler, G., *et al.*, Ethical challenges in contemporary psychiatry: An overview and an appraisal of possible strategies and research needs. *World Psychiatry*, 23, 3, 364–386, 2024.
34. Lustgarten, S.D., Garrison, Y.L., Sinnard, M.T., Flynn, A.W., Digital privacy in mental healthcare: Current issues and recommendations for technology use. *Curr. Opin. Psychol.*, 36, 25–31, 2020.
35. Lanz, J.G., de Montalvo Jååskelåinen, F., Parra, V.M., Barrutieta, L.H., Ethical and legal implications of digital mental health applications, 35, 143–155, 2024.
36. Wu, L., Data security and privacy considerations in mental health settings, in: *Chatbots and Mental Healthcare in Psychology and Psychiatry*, pp. 237–266, IGI Global, Hershey, Pennsylvania, USA, 2025.
37. Modi, T.B., Artificial intelligence ethics and fairness: A study to address bias and fairness issues in ai systems, and the ethical implications of ai applications. *Rev. Rev. Index J. Multi.*, 3, 2, 24–35, 2023.

38. Kinoshita, S., Cortright, K., Crawford, A., Mizuno, Y., Yoshida, K., Hilty, D., Guinart, D., Torous, J., Correll, C.U., Castle, D.J., *et al.*, Changes in telepsychiatry regulations during the covid-19 pandemic: 17 countries and regions' approaches to an evolving healthcare landscape. *Psychol. Med.*, 52, 13, 2606–2613, 2022.
39. Sethi, M., II, Kumar, R.C., Manjunatha, N., Kumar, C.N., Math, S.B., Mental health apps in india: Regulatory landscape and future directions. *BJPsych Int.*, 1–4, 2024.
40. Goktas, P. and Grzybowski, A., Shaping the future of healthcare: Ethical clinical challenges and pathways to trustworthy AI. *J. Clin. Med.*, 14, 5, 1605, 2025.
41. Balcombe, L. and De Leo, D., Human-computer interaction in digital mental health, in: *Informatics*, vol. 9, p. 14, MDPI, Basel, Switzerland, 2022.
42. Lu, H., Alhaskawi, A., Dong, Y., Zou, X., Zhou, H., Ezzi, S.H.A., Kota, V.G., Hasan Abdulla Hasan Abdulla, M., Abdalbary, S.A., Patient autonomy in medical education: Navigating ethical challenges in the age of artificial intelligence. *INQUIRY J. Health Care Organ. Provision Financ.*, 61, 00469580241266364, 2024.
43. Bond, R.R., Mulvenna, M.D., Potts, C., O'Neill, S., Ennis, E., Torous, J., Digital transformation of mental health services. *Npj Ment. Health Res.*, 2, 1, 13, 2023.
44. Mehmood, F., Mumtaz, N., Mehmood, A., Next-generation tools for patient care and rehabilitation: A review of modern innovations, in: *Actuators*, vol. 14, p. 133, MDPI, Basel, Switzerland, 2025.
45. H. kortas, Jemili, F., Korbaa, O., Early detection of mental health issues through machine learning: A comparative analysis of predictive models, 2024.
46. Han, K.M. and Kim, Y.K., Promising neural diagnostic biomarkers and predictors of treatment outcomes for psychiatric disorders: Novel neuroimaging approaches. *Prog. Neuro-psychopharmacol. Biol. Psychiatry*, 91, 1–3, 2019.
47. Benita, J., Jaswanth, S., Bhuvaneshwar, N., Yuvaraj, R., Narayana, Y.L., Phoenix: A conversational agent for emotional well-being and psychological support, in: *2025 International Conference on Multi-Agent Systems for Collaborative Intelligence (ICMSCI)*, IEEE, pp. 1137–1142, 2025.

48. Alhejaili, R., Wearable Technology for Mental Wellness Monitoring and Feedback, PhD thesis, Queen Mary University of London, 2023.
49. Robbins, R., Weaver, M.D., Sullivan, J.P., Quan, S.F., Gilmore, K., Shaw, S., Benz, A., Qadri, S., Barger, L.K., Czeisler, C.A., *et al.*, Accuracy of three commercial wearable devices for sleep tracking in healthy adults. *Sensors*, 24, 20, 6532, 2024.
50. de Aguiar, K.R., Cabelleira, M.D., Montezano, B.B., Jansen, K., de Azevedo Cardoso, T., Sleep alterations as a predictor of bipolar disorder among offspring of parents with bipolar disorder: A systematic review and meta-analysis, 2022.
51. Flanagan, K. and Saikia, M.J., Consumer-grade electroencephalogram and functional near-infrared spectroscopy neurofeedback technologies for mental health and wellbeing. *Sensors*, 23, 20, 8482, 2023.
52. lan Hong, T., Dave, Y., Khant, A., Verma, L., Chauhan, M., Parthasarathy, The future of personalized medicine and internet of things reshaping healthcare treatment plans and patient experiences. *J. Intell. Syst. Internet Things*, 14, 1, 2025.
53. Dobson, R., Li, L.L., Garner, K., Tane, T., McCool, J., Whittaker, R., *et al.*, The use of sensors to detect anxiety for in-the-moment intervention: Scoping review. *JMIR Mental Health*, 10, 1, e42611, 2023.
54. Rafika, A.S., Faturahman, A., Henry, B.N., Yulian, F.D., Hassan, M., AI-driven big data solutions for personalized healthcare: Analyzing patient data to improve treatment outcomes. *J. Comput. Sci. Technol. Appl.*, 2, 1, 36–45, 2025.
55. Siyadri, Y. and Deepak Akella, S.R., Advancing user-centric privacy: A comprehensive research roadmap for ethical and secure technology development. *i-Manager's J. Inf. Technol.*, 13, 3, 2024.
56. Hand, L.J., The role of telemedicine in rural mental health care around the globe. *Telemed. e-Health*, 28, 3, 285–294, 2022.
57. Bhatt, M. and Patel, M., Applications of virtual and augmented reality for health and well-being: Mental health treatment, in: *Modern Technology in Healthcare and Medical Education: Blockchain, IoT, AR, and VR*, pp. 129–140, IGI Global, Hershey, Pennsylvania, USA, 2024.
58. Oliinyk, A., Burdeinyi, A., Odintsov, A., Virtual reality exposure therapy protocol for post-traumatic stress disorder treatment in military veterans: Cross-cultural adaptation of virtual exposure therapy in Ukraine. *Mental Health*. 7, 118–128, 2024.

59. Chen, Y., Wang, T., Tan, Y., Li, D., Feasibility and effectiveness study of applying a hallucinogen harm reduction and integration model to a mindfulness thinking intervention using virtual reality: A randomized controlled trial. *Digit. Health*, 10, 20552076241249869, 2024.
60. Cheung, M., Xia, G., Xu, Z., A scoping review of somatosensory interaction design for mental health and well-being. *Acta Psychol.*, 253, 104641, 2025.
61. Bai, P., Application and mechanisms of internet-based cognitive behavioral therapy (icbt) in improving psychological state in cancer patients. *J. Cancer*, 14, 11, 1981, 2023.
62. Sharma, A. and Kaur, P., Tamper-proof multitenant data storage using blockchain. *Peer-to-peer Netw. Appl.*, 16, 1, 431–449, 2023.
63. Rai, B.K., Pcbehr: patient-controlled blockchain enabled electronic health records for healthcare 4.0. *Health Serv. Outcomes Res. Methodol.*, 23, 1, 80–102, 2023.
64. de Filippis, R. and Al Foysal, A., Blockchain brains: Pioneering AI, ml, and dlt solutions for healthcare and psychology. *Open Access Lib. J.*, 11, 12, 1–24, 2024.
65. Chapman, A.R., Breaking barriers: Bridging gaps in mental health literacy through digital innovation, 2025.
66. Thirupathi, L., Kaashipaka, V., Dhanaraju, M., Katakam, V., AI and IoT in mental health care: From digital diagnostics to personalized, continuous support, in: *Intelligent Systems and IoT Applications in Clinical Health*, pp. 271–294, IGI Global, Hershey, Pennsylvania, USA, 2025.
67. Sargiotis, D., Data security and privacy: Protecting sensitive information, in: *Data governance: a guide*, pp. 217–245, Springer, Cham, Switzerland, 2024.
68. Robinson, A., Flom, M., Forman-Hoffman, V.L., Histon, T., Levy, M., Darcy, A., Ajayi, T., Mohr, D.C., Wicks, P., Greene, C., *et al.*, Equity in digital mental health interventions in the united states: Where to next? *J. Med. Internet Res.*, 26, e59939, 2024.
69. Pasupuleti, M.K., Strategies for bridging the digital divide in rural and low-income communities, pp. 106–135, 2024.
70. Chauhan, S.N. and Vaidya, A.K., Challenges and opportunities. *Int. J. Nurs. Educ. Res.*, 12, 4, 2024.

71. Septiandri, A.A., Constantinides, M., Quercia, D., Weird icwsm: How western, educated, industrialized, rich, and democratic is social computing research?, arXiv preprint arXiv:2406.02090, 2024.
72. Aminabee, S., The future of healthcare and patient-centric care: Digital innovations, trends, and predictions, in: *Emerging Technologies for Health Literacy and Medical Practice*, pp. 240–262, IGI Global Scientific Publishing, Hershey, Pennsylvania, USA, 2024.
73. Deif, R. and Salama, M., Depression from a precision mental health perspective: Utilizing personalized conceptualizations to guide personalized treatments. *Front. Psychiatry*, 12, 650318, 2021.
74. Yasmeen, K., Nadeem, S., Imran, H., Bibi, A., Ahmad, T., Abbas, M.M., Jauhar, A.A., Enhancing treatment efficacy and user engagement in mental health care: Integrating ai into traditional therapeutic practices and addressing ethical considerations. *Social Sci. Rev. Arch.*, 2, 2, 66–79, 2024.
75. Hilty, D.M., Ahuja, S., Naslund, J.A., Crawford, A., Approaches to virtual care in underserved communities and settings: Bridging the behavioral health-care gap, in: *Virtual Mental Health Care for Rural and Underserved Settings*, pp. 101–129, Springer, Cham, Switzerland, 2022.
76. McClain, T., The wired couch: Untangling the promise and peril of telepsychiatry and mental health apps. *Psychiatr. News*, 59, 2024.
77. Mbanugo, O.J., Structural racism, healthcare policy, and their impact on health disparities among underserved populations in the united states.
78. Isa, A.K., Exploring digital therapeutics for mental health: AI-driven innovations in personalized treatment approaches. *World J. Adv. Res. Rev.*, 24, 2733–2749, 2024.
79. Paraschiv, E., Ianculescu, M., Gusatu, A., Constantin, V., Digital health platforms as educational tools: Enhancing self-management for patients with mental health conditions, in: *ICERI2024 Proceedings*, IATED, pp. 4338–4347, 2024.
80. Dey, S. and Singh, K., Early depression detection using modern ai techniques, in: *Advances in computational intelligence and robotics book series*, pp. 119–138, IGI Global, Hershey, Pennsylvania, USA, 2024.
81. Scala, J.J., Ganz, A.B., Snyder, M.P., Precision medicine approaches to mental health care. *Physiology*, 38, 2, 82–98, 2023.

82. Lee, K., Lee, T.C., Yefimova, M., Kumar, S., Puga, F., Azuero, A., Kamal, A., Bakitas, M.A., Wright, A.A., Demiris, G., *et al.*, Using digital phenotyping to understand health-related outcomes: a scoping review. *Int. J. Med. Inf.*, 174, 105061, 2023.
83. Isa, A.K., Exploring digital therapeutics for mental health: AI-driven innovations in personalized treatment approaches, 2024.
84. Altaf Dar, M., Maqbool, M., Ara, I., Zehravi, M., The intersection of technology and mental health: enhancing access and care. *Int. J. Adolesc. Med. Health*, 35, 5, 423–428, 2023.
85. Venture, M., Exploring Strategies for Social Impact in Cross-Sector Partnerships: A Multiple Case Study Approach, PhD thesis, Pepperdine University, 2024.
86. Katiyar, K., AI-based predictive analytics for patients' psychological disorder, in: *Predictive Analytics of Psychological Disorders in Healthcare: Data Analytics on Psychological Disorders*, pp. 37–53, Springer, Cham, Switzerland, 2022.
87. Ayhan, Y., The impact of artificial intelligence on psychiatry: Benefits and concerns-an assay from a disputed 'author'. *Turk. J. Psychiatry*, 34, 65–67, 2023.
88. Rostami, M., Abdi, M., Asadi, N.Z., Predicting the future of mental health interventions: The role of digital therapeutics. *J. Foresight Public Health*, 2, 2, 33–51, 2025.
89. Anikwe, C.V., Nweke, H.F., Ikegwu, A.C., Egwuonwu, C.A., Onu, F.U., Alo, U.R., Teh, Y.W., Mobile and wearable sensors for data-driven health monitoring system: State-of-the-art and future prospect. *Expert Syst. Appl.*, 202, 117362, 2022.
90. Thirupathi, L., Kaashipaka, V., Dhanaraju, M., Katakam, V., AI and IoT in mental health care, in: *Advances in medical technologies and clinical practice book series*, pp. 271–294, IGI Global, Hershey, Pennsylvania, USA, 2024.
91. Sherbini, D., The hidden cost of teletherapy, Chicago Policy Review (Online), 2023.
92. Olukayode, S.M., Arogundade, B., Adebanjo, A.O., Kalu, O.C., Digital mental health interventions and ai in therapy.
93. Kinkulkina, M.A. and Tikhonova, Y.G., Digital interventions in mental health: Challenges and perspectives. *Nacionalnoe Zdravoohranenie*, 4, 5–14, 2023.

94. Naslund, J.A., Mitchell, L.M., Joshi, U., Nagda, D., Lu, C., Economic evaluation and costs of telepsychiatry programmes: A systematic review. *J. Telemed. Telecare*, 28, 5, 311–330, 2022.
95. Glenthøj, L.B. and Faurholt-Jepsen, M., Editorial: Special issue on digital psychiatry, Acta Psychiatrica Scandinavica, 2024.
96. Kannan, K.D., Jagatheesaperumal, S.K., Kandala, R.N., Lotfaliany, M., Alizadehsanid, R., Mohebbi, M., Advancements in machine learning and deep learning for early detection and management of mental health disorder, arXiv preprint arXiv:2412.06147, 2024.
97. Dey, D.N.C., Mental health of adolescents and youth in india: A critical analysis in the era of AI, Available at SSRN 5056368, 2024.
98. Mabil-Atem, J.M., Gumuskaya, O., Wilson, R.L., Digital mental health interventions for the mental health care of refugees and asylum seekers: Integrative literature review. *Int. J. Ment. Health Nurs.*, 33, 4, 760–780, 2024.
99. Pham, K.T., Sheynin, J., Liberzon, I., A blueprint for next generation of clinical trials in precision psychiatry, pp. 83–91, Elsevier BV, 2024.
100. Mellman, T.A., Miller, A.L., Weissman, E.M., Crismon, M.L., Essock, S.M., Marder, S.R., Evidence-based pharmacologic treatment for people with severe mental illness: A focus on guidelines and algorithms. *Psychiatr. Serv.*, 52, 5, 619–625, 2001.
101. Lazarou, E. and Exarchos, T.P., Predicting stress levels using physiological data: Real-time stress prediction models utilizing wearable devices. *AIMS Neurosci.*, 11, 2, 76, 2024.
102. Ajayi, R., AI-powered innovations for managing complex mental health conditions and addiction treatments. *Int. Res. J. Mod. Eng. Technol. Sci.*, 7, 1, 87, 2025.
103. Diano, F., Sica, L.S., Ponticorvo, M., Empower psychotherapy with mhealth apps: The design of "safer", an emotion regulation application. *Information*, 14, 6, 308, 2023.
104. Sood, P., Tanwar, H., Singh, J., Ruhela, A.K., Gupta, N., Kumar, R., Revolutionizing customer service: An AI-powered chatbot approach using advanced nlp techniques, in: *2024 3rd Edition of IEEE Delhi Section Flagship Conference (DELCON)*, IEEE, pp. 1–5, 2024.
105. González Ramírez, M.L., García Vázquez, J.P., Rodríguez, M.D., Padilla-López, L.A., Galindo-Aldana, G.M., Cuevas-González, D., Wearables for stress management: A scoping review, in: *Healthcare*, vol. 11, p. 2369, MDPI, Basel, Switzerland, 2023.

106. Lee, M.-C., Chiang, S.-Y., Yeh, S.-C., Wen, T.-F., Study on emotion recognition and companion chatbot using deep neural network. *Multimedia Tools Appl.*, 79, 27, 19629–19657, 2020.
107. Cheng, Y., Lee, J., Qiao, J., Crisis communication in the age of AI: Navigating opportunities, challenges, and future horizons. *Media Crisis Commun.*, 172–194, 2024.
108. Grabowski, K., Rynkiewicz, A., Lassalle, A., Baron-Cohen, S., Schuller, B., Cummins, N., Baird, A., Podgórska-Bednarz, J., Pieniażek, A., Lucka, I., Emotional expression in psychiatric conditions: New technology for clinicians. *Psychiatry Clin. Neurosci.*, 73, 2, 50–62, 2019.
109. Aderinto, N., Olatunji, G., Muili, A., Kokori, E., Edun, M., Akinmoju, O., Yusuf, I., Ojo, D., A narrative review of non-invasive brain stimulation techniques in neuropsychiatric disorders: Current applications and future directions. *Egypt. J. Neurol. Psychiatr. Neurosurg.*, 60, 1, 50, 2024.
110. Dejene, B.K., Wearable smart textiles for mood regulation: A critical review of emerging technologies and their psychological impacts. *J. Ind. Text.*, 55, 15280837251314190, 2025.
111. Paraschiv, E.-A., Băjenaru, L., Petrache, C., Bica, O., Nicolau, D.-N., AI-driven neuro-monitoring: Advancing schizophrenia detection and management through deep learning and eeg analysis. *Future Internet*, 16, 11, 424, 2024.

Index

Also of Interest

Check out these other related titles from Scrivener Publishing

Artificial Intelligence and Machine Learning in Neurology, Edited by Abhishek Kumar, Pramod Singh Rathore, Sachin Ahuja, and Manoj Manuja, ISBN: 9781394389100. Unlock the future of brain health with this indispensable guide, which offers a comprehensive exploration of how artificial intelligence and machine learning are revolutionizing the diagnosis, treatment, and management of complex neurological disorders.

Artificial Intelligence in Healthcare for the Elderly, Edited by Sandeep Sharma, Preeti Nagrath, Bhawna Singla, and Joel J.P.C. Rodrigues, ISBN: 9781394275366. *Artificial Intelligence in Healthcare for the Elderly* provides valuable insights into how artificial intelligence can transform healthcare through personalized monitoring, ethical considerations, and real-world applications.

Design and Forecasting Models for Disease Management, Edited by Pijush Dutta, Sudip Mandal, Korhan Cengiz, Arindam Sadhu, and Gour Gopal Jana, ISBN: 9781394234042. The book provides an essential overview of AI techniques in disease management and how these computational methods can lead to further innovations in healthcare.

Smart Hospitals: 5G, 6G, and Moving Beyond Connectivity, Edited by Arun Kumar, Manoj Gupta, Sanjeev Sharma, Er. Himanshu Sharma, and Khursheed Aurangzeb, ISBN: 9781394275441. Discover the potential of 5G, 6G, and smart hospitals beyond connectivity in

Smart Hospitals: 5G, 6G, and Moving Beyond Connectivity and learn how these advancements are revolutionizing healthcare and the digital world.

Sustainable Nanomaterials for Treatment and Diagnosis of Infectious Diseases, Edited by Rajasekhar Chokkareddy, Suvardhan Kanchi and Gan G. Redhi, ISBN: 9781394200016. The book focuses on the design and novel synthetic routes of sustainable nanomaterials in diagnosing and treating infectious diseases offering potential benefits in terms of efficiency, biocompatibility, and environmental impact.

Federated Intelligent System for Healthcare: A Practical Guide, Edited by S. Rakesh Kumar, N. Gayathri and Seifedine Kadry, ISBN: 9781394271351. This practical guide gives valuable insights for integrating advanced technologies in healthcare, empowering researchers to effectively navigate and implement federated systems to enhance patient care.

Internet of Medicine for Smart Healthcare, Edited by Abhishek Kumar, Narayan Vyas, Pramod Singh Rathore, Abhineet Anand, and Pooja Dixit, ISBN: 9781394272235. This book provides in-depth explanations and discussions of the latest applications of AI, machine learning, and the Internet of Medicine, offering readers the cutting edge on this rapidly growing technology that has the potential to transform healthcare and improve patient outcomes.

Viral Vectors for Vaccine Delivery, Edited by Vivek Chavda and Vasso Apostolopoulos, ISBN: 9781394271535. The book is essential for anyone interested in vaccine development, as it highlights the unique advantages of viral vector vaccines in triggering robust, long-lasting immunity and provides an in-depth exploration of the technology and advancements shaping the future of healthcare.

Artificial Intelligence and Cybersecurity in Healthcare, Edited by Rashmi Agrawal, Pramod Singh Rathore, Ganesh Gopal Devarajan, and Rajiva Ranjan Divivedi, ISBN: 9781394229796. *Artificial Intelligence and Cybersecurity in Healthcare* offers a vital exploration of the intersection of artificial intelligence and cybersecurity within healthcare Cyber Physical Systems, equipping readers with knowledge on how to navigate the transformative yet complex technological landscape shaping modern patient care and data protection.

Explainable Artificial Intelligence in the Healthcare Industry, Edited by Abhishek Kumar, T. Ananth Kumar, Prasenjit Das, Chetan Sharma, and Ashutosh Kumar Dubey, ISBN: 9781394249268. Discover the essential insights and practical applications of explainable AI in healthcare that will empower professionals and enhance patient trust with Explainable AI in Healthcare, a must-have resource for anyone looking to navigate the future of medical practices with confidence.

Role of Flavonoids in Chronic Metabolic Diseases: From Bench to Clinic, Edited by Neeraj Mishra, Sumel Ashique, B.H. Jaswanth Gowda, Arshad Farid, Ashish Garg, ISBN: 9781394238040. This comprehensive volume covers the entire field of flavonoids by explaining their complex functions in reducing chronic metabolic illnesses, from the early stages of laboratory research to the development of therapeutic uses.

Printed and bound by CPI Group (UK) Ltd, Croydon, CR0 4YY

17/09/2026

14964285-0001